HEPATITIS C VIRUS :
NEW DIAGNOSTIC TOOLS

British Library Cataloguing in Publication Data
A catalogue record for this book is available from the British Library.

ISBN : 2-7420-0052-6

Éditions John Libbey Eurotext
127, avenue de la République, 92120 Montrouge, France
Tel. : (1) 46.73.06.60

John Libbey and Company Ltd
13, Smiths Yard, Summerley Street,
London SW18 4HR, England.
Tel. : (1) 947.27.77

John Libbey CIC
Via L. Spallanzani, 11
00161, Rome, Italy.
Tel. : (06) 862.289

© 1994, John Libbey Eurotext, Paris

Il est interdit de reproduire intégralement ou partiellement le présent ouvrage — loi du 11 mars 1957 — sans autorisation de l'éditeur ou du Centre Français du Copyright, 6 *bis*, rue Gabriel-Laumain, 75010 Paris.

HEPATITIS C VIRUS : NEW DIAGNOSTIC TOOLS

Groupe Français d'Études Moléculaires des Hépatites
GEMHEP

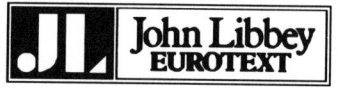

Contents

List of contributors	VII
Foreword D. Dhumeaux	IX

1. **Hepatitis C virus genetic variability : clinical implications**
   C. Bréchot 1

2. **Significance of indeterminate second generation RIBA and resolution by third generation RIBA**
   J.M. Pawlotsky 17

3. **Role of liver disease and hepatitis C virus infection in the pathogenesis of mixed cryoglobulinemia**
   L. Musset, F. Lunel 29

4. **HCV genotypes and genotyping methods**
   L. Stuyver 39

5. **Multicentre quality control of hepatitis C virus RNA polymerase chain reaction**
   J.J. Lefrère and the GEMHEP 49

6. **Branched DNA (bDNA) quantitation of hepatitis C viral RNA in patient sera**
   J. Kolberg, R. Sanchez-Pescador, J. Detmer, M. Collins, P. Sheridan, P. Neuwald, J. Wilber, P. Dailey, M. Urdea 57

7. **Specific detection of HCV RNA using NASBA™ as a diagnostic tool**
   P. Sillekens, W. Kok, B. van Gemen, P. Lens, H. Huisman, T. Cuypers, T. Kievits 71

8. **Detection of HCV RNA in serum using a single-tube, single enzyme PCR in combination with a colorimetric microwell assay**
   L. Wolfe, S. Tamatsukuri, C. Sayada, J.C. Ryff 83

9. **Quantitation of serum hepatitis C virus RNA by branched DNA amplification and distibution of HCV genotypes in anti-HCV positive blood donors**
   P. Marcellin, M. Martinot-Peignoux, J. Gournay, J.P. Benhamou, S. Erlinger 95

10. **Viremia, a more interesting factor than HCV genotype in chronic hepatitis C for predictive response to alpha-interferon therapy**
M.A. Thelu, V. Barlet, M. Cohard, J.M. Seigneurin, J.P. Zarski 103

Conclusion
S. Erlinger 107

List of contributors

Barlet V., Laboratoire de Virologie Médicale Moléculaire, CHU, Grenoble, France.
Benhamou J.P., Service d'Hépatologie et INSERM U24, Hôpital Beaujon, Clichy, France.
Bréchot C., INSERM U370 and Liver Unit, CHU Necker, Paris, et Laboratoire Hybridotest (CBMS), Institut Pasteur, Paris, France.
Cohard M., Laboratoire de Virologie Médicale Moléculaire et Service d'Hépato-gastro-entérologie, CHU, Grenoble, France.
Collins M., Chiron Corporation, Emeryville, CA, USA.
Cuypers T., Central Laboratory of the Netherlands Red Cross Blood Transfusion Service, Plesmanlaan 125, 1066 CX, Amsterdam, The Netherlands.
Dailey P., Chiron Corporation, Emeryville, CA, USA.
Detmer J., Chiron Corporation, Emeryville, CA, USA.
Dhumeaux D., Service d'Hépatologie et de Gastroentérologie, Hôpital Henri-Mondor, 94010 Créteil, France.
Erlinger S., Service d'Hépatologie et INSERM U24, Hôpital Beaujon, Clichy, France.
van Gemen B., Organon Teknika, Boseind 15, 5280 AB Boxtel, The Netherlands.
Gournay J., Service d'Hépatologie et INSERM U24, Hôpital Beaujon, Clichy, France.
Huisman H., Central Laboratory of the Netherlands Red Cross Blood Transfusion Service, Plesmanlaan 125, 1066 CX, Amsterdam, The Netherlands.
Kievits T., Organon Teknika, Boseind 15, 5280 AB Boxtel, The Netherlands.
Kok W., Organon Teknika, Boseind 15, 5280 AB Boxtel, The Netherlands.
Kolberg J., Chiron Corporation, Emeryville, CA, USA.
Lefrère J.J., Institut National de Transfusion Sanguine, Hôpital Saint-Antoine, Paris, France.
Lens P., Organon Teknika, Boseind 15, 5280 AB Boxtel, The Netherlands.
Lunel F., Service de Bactériologie-Virologie, Groupe Hospitalier Pitié-Salpêtrière, 43-47, bd de l'Hôpital, 75651 Paris Cedex 13, France.
Marcellin P., Service d'Hépatologie et INSERM U24, Hôpital Beaujon, Clichy, France.
Martinot-Peignoux M., Service d'Hépatologie et INSERM U24, Hôpital Beaujon, Clichy, France.
Musset L., Service d'Immunochimie, Groupe Hospitalier Pitié-Salpêtrière, 43-47, bd de l'Hôpital, 75651 Paris Cedex 13, France.
Neuwald P., Chiron Corporation, Emeryville, CA, USA.
Pawlotsky J.M., Department of Bacteriology and Virology, Hôpital Henri Mondor, Université Paris XII, 94010 Créteil, France.

Ryff J.C., Department of International Clinical Research, Hoffmann-La Roche, Basel, Switzerland.
Sanchèz-Pescador R., Chiron Corporation, Emeryville, CA, USA.
Sayada C., Roche Diagnostics, Paris, France.
Seigneurin J.M., Laboratoire de Virologie Médicale Moléculaire, CHU, Grenoble, France.
Sheridan P., Chiron Corporation, Emeryville, CA, USA.
Sillekens P., Organon Teknika, Boseind 15, 5280 AB Boxtel, The Netherlands.
Stuyver L., Innogenetics NV, Industriepark 7, box 4, B-9052, Gent, Belgium.
Tamatsukuri S., Nippon Roche, Tokyo, Japan.
Thelu M.A., Laboratoire de Virologie Médicale Moléculaire, CHU, Grenoble, France.
Urdea M., Chiron Corporation, Emeryville, CA, USA.
Wilber J., Chiron Corporation, Emeryville, CA, USA.
Wolfe L., Roche Molecular System, Branchburg, NJ, USA.
Zarski J.P., Laboratoire de Virologie Médicale Moléculaire et Service d'Hépato-gastro-entérologie, CHU, Grenoble, France.

Foreword

The French group for molecular study of hepatitis (called GEM-HEP) is an association of virologists, transfusionists and hepatologists. This group was created in 1991 upon the onset of the first multicentre quality control study of hepatitis C virus RNA polymerase chain reaction in France. The aim of this group was to pool efforts for the development and evaluation of new technologies of molecular biology in viral hepatology. Since its birth, the GEMHEP had organized two meetings : the first in Paris in 1991, the second one also in Paris (though this could change !) in November 1993.

This book contains the lectures of the last meeting which dealt with all the recent progresses in the diagnostic techniques developed for the presently most popular hepatotropic agent, hepatitis C virus. These included serological assays, amplification procedures, RNA quantitation, genotyping and serotyping, all topics covered by European specialists.

Fort the hepatologist, the hepatitis C virus is a fascinating but time-consuming problem. I (scientifically) evaluated that in 1993, each day, a mean of three papers was published on it. The resulting mass of information makes that good meetings synthetizing recent and as yet unpublished data are welcome. I attended the November meeting of GEMHEP, and it was actually welcome.

Daniel DHUMEAUX
Hôpital Henri-Mondor, Créteil, France

1

Hepatitis C virus genetic variability : clinical implications

C. BRÉCHOT

*INSERM U-370 and Liver Unit, CHU Necker, Paris, France.
Laboratoire Hybridotest (CBMS), Institut Pasteur, Paris, France.*

Hepatitis C virus

Hepatitis C virus (HCV) has been identified in 1988 and is now recognised as the major etiologic agent of NonA-NonB [1-8] hepatitis. An efficient cell culture system for this virus, as well as convincing electron microscopic pictures have however still not be obtained. Thus, most of our knowledge is based on nucleotide and amino acid sequence analyses. HCV is an enveloped positively stranded RNA virus. The size of its RNA is variable among different isolates but averages 10 kilobases (kb). Its genomic organisation shares significant similarities with that of the pestiviruses although only limited homology can be shown at the nucleotidic level (Figure 1). The density of the HCV serum particles is highly variable, ranging from 1.1 to 1.17 g/ml ; this might be related in part to the association of the virus to macromolecules such as lipoproteins as well as to the presence of circulating immune complexes containing the viral particles. It is also not known how complete and defective particles are distributed [9].

The viral RNA is first translated into a large polyprotein (around 3,000 aminoacids) which is secondarily processed in structural (capsid and envelope) and non structural proteins. A number of studies are now investigating the processing pathways involved in the cleavage of the polyprotein. The function of the non structural proteins is still in part unclear ; NS3 however encodes in its N-terminal part for a serine

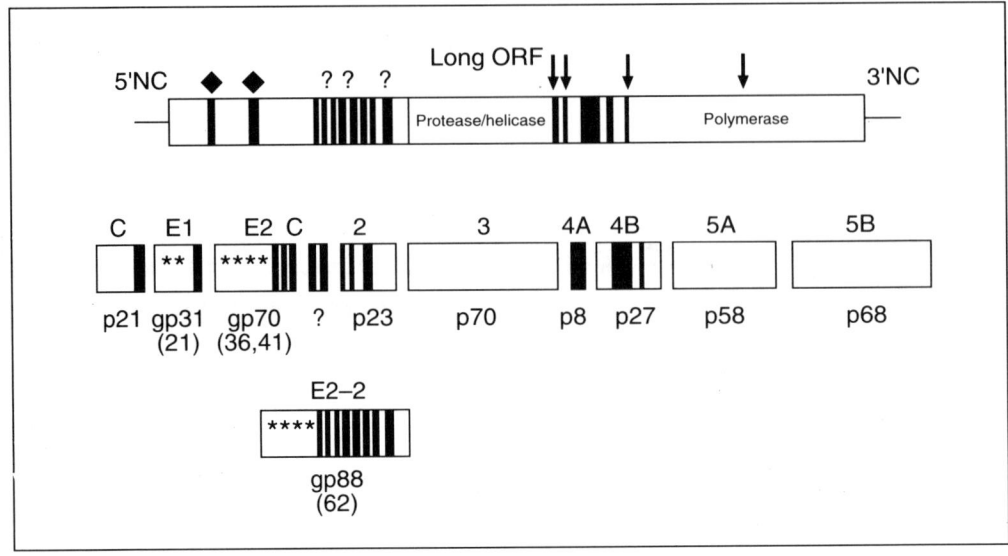

Figure 1. HCV polyprotein synthesis and processing (Grakoui et al., J Virology 1993, 67 : 2832).

proteinase which cleaves at the NS3/NS4 and NS4/NS5 junctions. The C-terminal part of the NS3 protein also shows helicase activity, likely involved in the replication of the viral RNA. An additional, distinct, serine proteinase activity has recently been described which is also encoded by NS3. Host signal peptidases are also involved and cleave the capsid and envelope proteins E1 and E2 [9, 11-14].

The mechanisms of HCV RNA replication are still poorly understood ; this is due to the fact that, as mentioned earlier, there is presently no efficient cell culture system [15-22] ; in addition there are difficulties to obtain complete reconstruction of full length cDNAs which would lead after transfection in eucaryotic cells to the synthesis of mature viral particles. Negative HCV RNA strands have been however detected which likely are intermediates in the replication cycle of the virus ; they have been identified in infected liver and mononuclear blood cells. Surprisingly they can also be identified, although in a much less amount, in the serum : it has been hypothesized that they would circulate in nucleoproteic complexes and not in complete viral particles [23]. There are no DNA intermediates in the HCV replication and thus no integration of HCV genome. Finally the NS5 encoded protein shows the RGD conserved motif among RNA polymerase and likely acts as an RNA dependent RNA polymerase. *In vitro* expression of some of the viral proteins has been obtained : the capsid and the E1 and E2 proteins have been expressed, using in particular the vaccinia and Baculovirus models [9, 24, 25].

The 5' extremity of the viral genome is not translated and thus referred to as the 5' non coding sequence [26]. It shows secondary, hairpin, structures and an internal ribosome entry site (IRES) [13, 26] which allows translation of the polyprotein. The length of the 3' non translated part of the HCV RNA has yet only been characterized in detail for a few HCV RNA molecules. It is however variable as well as its nucleotidic sequence. Several evidences suggest that this 3' extremity might play an important role for HCV RNA replication.

HCV, as an RNA virus, shows a marked genetic variability (around 10^{-3} substitutions per site and per year) [27-38]. This is likely related to infidelity of the RNA replication by the RNA dependent-RNA polymerase. This figure has been evaluated by two complementaries approaches : 1) analysis of serial serum samples from infected humans and chimpanzees with a long time follow up available and 2) comparison of the nucleotide sequence from a high number of HCV RNA molecules purified from the sera of individuals from various geographical areas (Table I).

Table I. Genetic variability of HCV.

	HCV infected patient (H) (13 years follow-up)		HCV infected chimpanzee (C) (8.2 years follow-up)	
	Nucleotides changes		Aminoacids changes	
	H	C	H	C
5'UTR	0.7 %	0	NA	NA
Core	1.4 %	0.9 %	1.4 %	1 %
E1	2.4 %	1.7 %	1.3 %	3.1 %
E2/NS1	4.6 %	2.2 %	7.2 %	4.3 %
NS2	3 %	1.7 %	1.8 %	0.7 %
NS3	1.9 %	1.1 %	1.2 %	0.5 %
NS4	NT	0.3 %	NA	0.2 %
NS5	1.9 %	1.1 %	1.5 %	1.3 %
3'UTR	NT	2.4 %	NT	NA
Mutation rate =	$\begin{bmatrix} 1.92 \times 10^{-3} \text{ base substitution / site / year (H)} \\ 1.44 \times 10^{-3} \text{ base subtitution / site / year (C)} \end{bmatrix}$			

Ogata et al. Proc Natl Acad Sci USA 1991 ; 88 : 3392.
Okamoto et al. Virology 1992 ; 190 : 894-899.

Clearly the extent of variability markedly varies from one part of the viral genome to the other. The 5' non coding region is highly conserved among the different HCV RNA types although mutations are also present in this domain. The capsid encoding region is, albeit to a less extent, conserved among different isolates. In contrast, the envelope proteins E1 and E2 show much more significant divergences; there are in particular « Hypervariable regions » located at the N-terminal part of E2. The higher aminoacid variability than nucleotidic variability in the E2 region suggests that the protein has low structural constraint and is subjected to rapid selection under various pressures (some evidences suggest that the mutation rate might be higher at the acute phase of HCV infection than later on in the chronic course of viral infection). Comparisons between nucleotide and aminoacid changes indicate that, for in these domains, most of the nucleotidic mutations lead to a change in aminoacids (non synonymous mutations). The non structural NS2, NS3 and NS4 proteins are less divergent than the NS5 domain which shows a number of mutations from one type to the other.

With the availability of numerous HCV RNA sequences, an attempt has been made to classify these HCV RNAs in different types and subtypes. Phylogenetic trees have been proposed. This is still a controversial issue since these classifications have been based for most HCV RNA molecules examined, on partial sequences. Thus classifications have been suggested from the comparison of the 5' non coding [39] or the NS5 sequences [40]. Recent data obtained with the envelope encoding sequences might however differ [28]. In any case, classification from partial HCV RNA sequences can only be reliable in the absence of evidence for recombination between different HCV types and, so far, this condition seems to be met (Table II).

Thus, genotypes of HCV have been individualized, HCV RNAs among a given type differing in their nucleotide sequence by less than 15 % and being referred to as « subtypes ». The number of HCV types and subtypes is still increasing and at least 12 genotypes might exist. A major point to be underlined is that, although some HCV genotypes are clearly most prevalent in some geographical areas, there is a mixing in a given country of various types and subtypes. The comparison between four different proposed classifications is shown in Table I. As mentioned earlier there is not a definitive agreement on this issue. In the following sections however, we will use a combination of the classifications proposed by Okamoto *et al.* and Stuyvers and Simmonds *et al.*

Table II. HCV genotypes — Classification

Chiron	Enomoto	Okamoto	Simmonds	
I	KPT	I	1	a
II	K1	II		b
nc	nc	nc		c
III	K2a	III	2	a
III	K2b	IV		b
nc	nc	nc		c
IV	nc	V	3	a
IV		VI		b
nc	nc	nc	4a	
V	nc	nc	5a	
nc		nc	6a	

Cha (PNAS 1992 ; 89 : 7144) ; Okamoto (J Gen Virol 1992 ; 73 : 673). [41].
Simmonds (J Gen Virol 1993 ; 74 : 661) ; Enomoto (BBRC 1990 ; 170 : 1021).

The viral genome is in fact present as a mixed population of closely, yet heterogeneous, related HCV RNA molecules. Such molecules are often designated as quasispecies. They include both replication competent and defective viruses which might modulate the viral infection and favor persistent HCV infection. It has been in fact suggested that, at least in some patients, the majority of the circulating HCV RNA molecules might be defective. This observation should be taken in account when considering the impact of HCV genetic variability.

Clinical implications of HCV genetic variability

In view of the mixing in a given country of different HCV types, several studies have investigated whether or not some HCV genotypes might show particular clinicopathological features. There are however a number of difficulties to be underlined in these studies :

Technical limitations : rapid procedures are clearly mandatory to investigate these issues on a large scale. Thus, procedures based on the polymerase chain reaction (PCR) have been set up. Schematically three complementary approaches have been used :

1. Digestion of the amplified products with restriction enzymes, thus generating a restriction fragment length polymorphism (RLP) [29, 39-41]. This technique is however difficult to use on a semi-routine basis and does not distinguish precisely in fact between the most relevant genotypes (see below). This is particularly important for identifying genotype II (1b).

2. Use of genotype specific primers for performing the PCR. This assay has allowed a number of studies to be conducted [42, 43]. However, some HCV RNA isolates cannot be classified by this assay among types which are heterogeneous and for which only a limited number of sequences are available to define efficient, type-specific primers (this is in particular the case for genotype III (2a)).

3. Hybridization of HCV RNA sequences with type-specific probes. This approach appears to be now reliable and rapid. It generally allows proper classification in the most prevalent genotypes [44].

It is noteworthy that the efficiency of these different assays for identifying mixed HCV infections is still debated. Although infections by different HCV types seems infrequent (5 % to 10 %), its prevalence is much higher (20 % ?) in some polytransfused patients (such as hemophiliacs [45] and hemodialyzed subjects).

4. It is also noteworthy that, beside genotyping, it is possible to precisely analyze RNA molecules present in a given infected subjects by amplification of an hypervariable sequence [30, 46, 47] (Table III).

Table III. Precise identification of HCV strain. Analysis of an hypervariable nucleotide sequence : E_1 or E_2/NS_1

1. **Demonstration of reinfection of liver graft by the original HCV.**
   Feray et al. J Clin Invest 1992 ; 89 : 1361.
2. **Mother to Child and sexual transmission.**
   Inoue et al. Nature 1991 ; 353 : 609 (Enveloppe),
   Kao et al. J Infect Dis 1992 ; 166 : 900 (NS_3).
3. **Selection of HCV RNA molecules during the course of HCV infection.**
   Weiner et al. Proc Natl Acad Sci USA 1992 ; 89 : 3468.
   Kumar U et al. J Infect Dis 1993 ; 167 : 3
4. **Evaluation of protective immunity.**
   Farci et al. Science 1992 ; 258 : 135.

Clinical bias

As usual, clinical bias are important to consider and the preliminary observations were based on small series and did not take in account confounding factors such as age and duration of the viral infection. It is also important to clearly distinguish between non responders, relapsers and long term responders to treatment by interferon alpha.

Clinicopathological correlations

A number of investigations have been reported, mostly however at the present time in abstracts.

1. There is a distinct repartition of HCV types according to the geographical areas. HCV II (1b) is highly prevalent in Japan (70-80 %) and in Europe (50-70 %). Only scarce data are presently available in the US but they also suggest a high prevalence of HCV II (1b). Other prevalent HCV types in these areas are type I (1a), III (2a) and IV (2b). In contrast there are marked divergences in Africa and middle East : in particular we and others have shown a high prevalence of HCV type 4 in central Africa and Egypt. It is however important to note that genotypes such as type 4 and 5 can in fact also be identified in some European infected subjects.

2. Genotype II (1b) is associated to a low response to interferon alpha and beta.

This has been first suggested in Japan in studies where other factors were not however included in the analysis. Recent studies in Europe conducted in Benelux and France (our work) have recently confirmed, using multivariate analysis, that infection by HCV type II (1b) is an independent prognostic factor for a non response or relapse after therapy. In contrast, genotype III (2a) was shown in Japan to be associated to a good response to IFN (Figure 2) [48-51].

These data are obviously of major importance since they might lead to modify the therapeutic strategies according to the HCV genotype.

Much work is however needed to expand these observations and in particular on the features of other, less represented, genotypes (such as 2a (III), 2b (IV), 3 (V), 4, 5, etc.).

3. Association of some genotypes to severe liver disease.

Two studies (in Japan and Italy) have led to hypothesize, from a limited number of patients examined, that HCV II (1b) might be highly prevalent in patients with cirrhosis and in those with HCC [52-54].

Other studies in Japan (presented as abstracts in the Tokyo meeting in May 1993) also showed a higher prevalence of HCV II (1b) in subjects with cirrhosis than in those with chronic hepatitis ; the differences were however not significant and other variables were not taken into account.

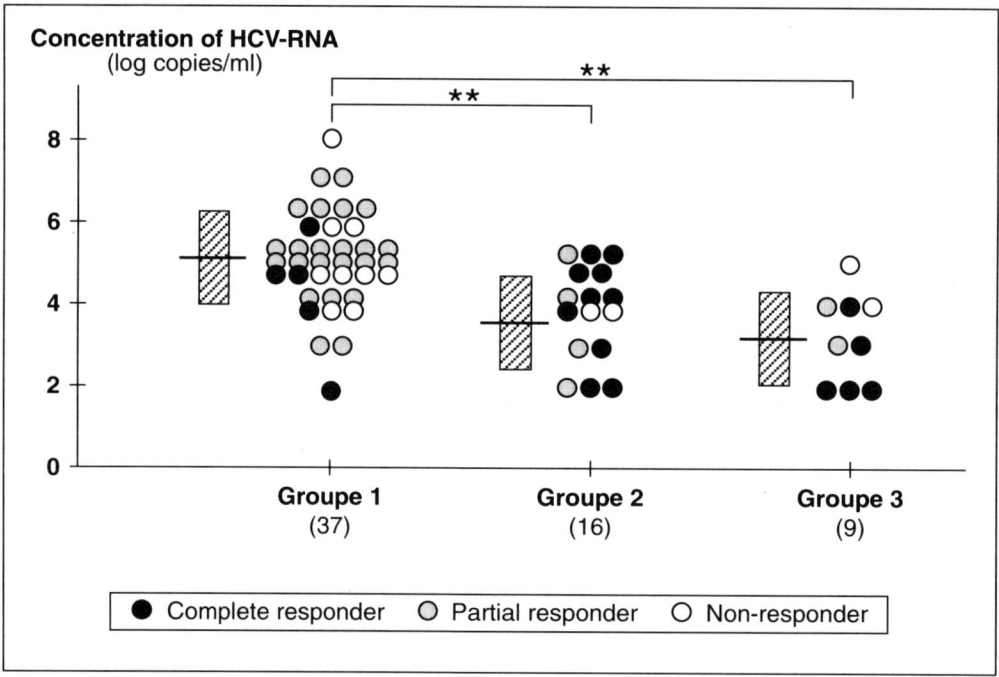

Figure 2. HCV RNA genotype and response to inferferon α (Yoshioka *et al.*, Hepatology, 1992, 16 : 293).

To adress this issue we have used recently two complementary approaches :

a) We analyzed liver transplant recipients grafted for HCV related cirrhosis. Previous studies from our group and others [46] have shown that at least 80 % of these liver grafts are reinfected by the original HCV strain. Comparison of the outcome of HCV infection on the liver graft showed that infection by HCV II (1b) led more frequently to acute and chronic hepatitis than « non II (1b) » genotypes. Thus, in a study where duration of the viral infection is by definition strictly controlled, there was direct evidence for a distinct cytopathogenic effect of HCV II (1b).

b) We have also investigated HCV genotypes in three different groups of patients with either chronic hepatitis, cirrhosis or HCC. Our results showed :

- The significantly higher prevalence of HCV II (1b) in patients with cirrhosis (with or without associated HCC), compared to these with chronic hepatitis (80 % vs 50 %).
- The correlation between the relative prevalence of HCV genotypes and age and duration of the viral infection : prevalence of HCV II (1b) was around 80 % in subjects above 60 years old or with a viral infection lasting for more than 15 years. In contrast, HCV II (1b) was much less prevalent in patients under 30 years old or with a disease duration under 5 years (around 30 %). Thus there is a marked decline in the relative prevalence of HCV II (1b) over the last decades and an increase in more recently introduced HCV types, likely due to new modes of transmission such as intravenous drug injections.
- As described in Benelux, genotype II (1b) was an independent prognostic factor for a low response to interferon alpha, being rarely observed in long term responders.

Therefore, altogether, the available data indicate that genotyping does provide clinically relevant informations.

4. The clinical impact of HCV genetic variability might be also explored in the future by serological assays. Peptides have been synthesized from different HCV sequences which allow to detect specific antibodies in infected subjects and to grossly distinguish between groups of HCV types. This approach is promising but has to be further refined [5].

5. The complexity of the viral population might also have implications for the evolution of HCV infection following treatment by interferon alpha : it has been indeed hypothesized that a mixing of different related HCV RNA molecules in a patient before treatment might indicate a further absence of response to therapy. One may envisage that selection of HCV RNA molecules might be favored by the treatment, with the emergence of variants potentially escaping the immune response and/or the antiviral effect of the drug [30, 47, 55, 56].

HCV genotypes : biological features

The hypothesis that different HCV types might have particular pattern of response to IFN and, possibly, lead to a different course of the viral infection, raises the issue of the mechanisms involved :

1. HCV types might show different rates of replication and thus different levels of viremia [49, 50, 57, 58].

This possibility has been investigated by using either « quantitative » RT-PCR or, more recently, the branched chain DNA assay (bDNA) [10]. One study in Japan showed higher mean HCV RNA levels in patients infected by HCV II (1b) as compared to these infected by HCV III (2a). There are indeed now solid evidence for HCV III (2a) being associated to low HCV RNA levels and good response to IFN treatment.

In our hand, however, when comparing HCV II (1b) to all « non II (1b) » types, we failed to evidence a significant difference in HCV viremia in transplant as well as non transplant recipients. In fact HCV viremia was, in a multivariate analysis, an independent prognostic factor for response to IFN, patients with low serum HCV RNA being more likely to be long term responders. Thus, it is likely that some HCV types do have a particular rate of replication but this does not account for all features described in the previous sections.

2. Some HCV types might show a particular interplay whith the host immune system. As described in the section 1, the envelope proteins (mostly E2) exhibit a marked variability. Follow up studies are consistent with these aminoacid changes being due to selection by the immune response of some HCV RNA molecules. Evidence has been indeed presented for the presence in the hypervariable region located in E2 of B and T cells epitopes. Antibodies to these domains have been identified in infected human and chimpanzees. Further studies will now explore with or not some HCV types (such as III (2a) for example) might induce specific immune response from the host.

3. Finally it is also important to realize that, in pestiviruses [14], modifications in the processing of the viral proteins might lead to enhanced cytopathic effects of the viral investigation. There are presently however no data concerning HCV to substantiate this hypothesis.

Genetic variability of HCV : implications for prevention of the viral infection

The sequence of the N-terminal part of the E2 encoding domain of HCV is highly variable and thus has been referred to as the « Hypervariable region 1 » (HVR1). This region varies from one patient to the other and during the acute to chronic transition phase, and subsequently the chronic course of HCV infection [30]. In some responders, these aminoacid changes correlated with exacerbation of hepatitis [48]. Antibodies to the HVR1 have been detected in infected subjects ; they appeared sequentially, being directed to new variants of the original HCV RNA molecules [55]. These observations are consistent with a selection of HCV RNA variants over time capable to escape to neutralizing the antibodies. Recent evidence in support of this hypothesis comes from *in vitro* and *in vivo* studies :

1. It has been recently demonstrated that a T-lymphocytic human cell line [58, 59] can be infected by HCV inocula and that there is a correlation between the *in vivo* and *in vitro* infectiosity titers. Using this system, antibodies preventing infection of the cells by an HCV inoculum (thus referred to as neutralizing antibodies) can be identified in HCV infected patients ; however their titer will decline over years.

2. Recent *in vivo* experiments also indicate the possibility to prevent infection of chimpanzees by neutralizing infection by an HCV inoculum with serum collected early in the course of HCV infection [58]. In contrast previous studies showed the possibility to reinfect chimpanzees, after apparent recovery of an HCV infection, with the same HCV isolate as well as an heterologous strain [58].

Therefore, altogether the current evidences indicate that neutralizing antibodies might be present early in the course of HCV infection and disappear later on. Expression, using vaccinia virus or Baculovirus, of the envelope proteins E1 and E2, associated in multimeric complexes, has been obtained. Injection to chimpanzees yields synthesis of antibodies which offer partial protection to the same HCV stain used for expressing the HCV proteins. The implication of these findings for passive and active immunotherapy will be however markedly hampered by the marked variability of these epitopes.

Finally it should be also emphasized that the role of the cellular immune response [60] to the virus is also likely to be a major factor to be considered for further analysis [61-63].

Conclusions

There is now evidences to support the hypothesis that the genetic variability of HCV has clinically significant impact. Much work has to be done to standardize the genotyping assays and the classification. It will be also important to further investigate the changing epidemiology of these HCV types over time and their association to some modes of transmission.

On a practical basis, all the data presented indicate that determining the genotype of HCV might be, together with the estimation of HCV viremia, part of management of HCV infected subjects.

References

1. Paterlini P, Driss F, Nalpas B, et al. Persistence of hepatitis B and hepatitis C viral genomes in primary liver cancers from HBsAg-negative patients : a study from a low-endemic area. Hepatology 1993 ; 17 : 20-9.
2. Saito I, Miyamura T, Ohbayashi A, et al. Hepatitis C virus infection is associated with the development of hepatocellular carcinoma. Proc Natl Acad Sci USA 1990 ; 87 : 6547-9.
3. Lok ASF, Ma OCK. Hepatitis B virus replication in Chinese patients with hepatocellular carcinoma. Hepatology 1990 ; 12 : 582-8.
4. Raimondo G, Burk R, et al. Interrupted replication of hepatitis B virus in liver tissue of HBsAg carriers with hepatocellular carcinoma. Virology 1988 ; 166 : 103-12.
5. Yuki N, Hayashi N, Kamada T. HCV viraemia and liver injury in symptom-free blood donors. Lancet 1993 ; 342 : 444.
6. Davis G, Balart L, Schiff E, Lindsay K, Bodenheimer H, Perrillo R. Treatment of chronic hepatitis C with recombinant interferon alpha. A multicenter randomized, controlled trial. N Engl J Med 1989 ; 321 : 1501-6.
7. Di Bisceglie A, Martin P, Kassianides C, et al. Recombinant interferon alfa therapy for chronic hepatitis C. A randomized, double-blind, placebo-controlled trial. N Engl J Med 1989 ; 321 : 1506-10.
8. Lau J, Davis G, Kniffen J, et al. Significance of serum hepatitis C virus RNA levels in chronic hepatitis C. Lancet 1993 ; 341 : 1501-4.
9. Matsuura Y, Miyamura T. The molecular biology of hepatitis C virus. Virology 1993 ; 4 : 297-304.
10. Urdea M, Horn T, Fultz T, et al. Branched DNA amplification multimers for the sensitive, direct detection of human hepatitis viruses. Nucl Acid Res 1991 ; 24 : 197-200.
11. Grakoui A, McCourt DW, Wychowski C, Feinstone SM. A second hepatitis C virus-enclosed proteinase. Proc Natl Acad Sci USA 1993 ; 90 : 10583-7.

12. Choo QL, Richman K, Han J, et al. Genetic organization and diversity of the hepatitis C virus. Proc Natl Acad Sci 1991 ; 88 : 2451-5.
13. Tsukiyama-Kohara T, Iizuka N, Kohara M, Nomoto A. Internal ribosome entry site within hepatitis C virus RNA. J Virol 1992 ; 66 : 1476-83.
14. Collett M, Moennig V, Horzinek M. Recent advances in pestivirus research. J Gen Virol 1989 ; 70 : 253-66.
15. Iacovacci S, Sargiacomo M, Parolini I, Ponzetto A, Peschle C, Carloni G. Replication and multiplication of hepatitis C virus genome in human foetal liver cells. Res Virol 1993 ; 144 : 275-9.
16. Bouffard P, Hayashi PH, Acevedo R, Levy N, Zeldis JB. Hepatitis C virus is detected in a monocyte : macrophage subpopulation of peripheral blood mononuclear cells of infected patients. J Infect Dis 1992 ; 166 : 1276-80.
17. Sherman KE, O'Brien J, Gutierrez AG, Harrison S, Urdea M, Neuwald P, Wilber J. Quantitative evaluation of hepatitis C virus RNA in patients with concurrent human immunodeficiency virus infections. J Clin Microbiol 1993 ; 2679-82.
18. Mocarski ES, Bonyhadi M, Salimi S, McCune JM, Kaneshima H. Human cytomegalovirus in a SCID-hu mouse : Thymic epithelial cells are prominent targets of viral replication. Proc Natl Acad Sci USA 1993 ; 90 : 104-8.
19. Tyor WR, Power C, Gendelman HE, Markham RB. A model of human immunodeficiency virus encephalitis in scid mice. Proc Natl Acad Sci USA 1993 ; 90 : 8658-62.
20. Müller HM, Pfaff E, Goeser T, Kallinowski B, Solbach C, Theilmann L. Peripheral blood leukocytes serve as a possible extrahepatic site for hepatitis C virus replication. J Gen Virol 1993 ; 74 : 669-76.
21. Zignego AL, Macchia D, Monti M, Thiers V, Mazzeti M, Foschi M, Maggi E, Romagnani S, Gentilini P, Bréchot C. Infection of peripheral mononuclear blood cells by hepatitis C virus. J Hepatol 1992 ; 15 : 382-6.
22. Qian C, Camps J, Maluenda MD, Civeira MP, Prieto J. Replication of hepatitis C virus in peripheral blood mononuclear cells. Effect of alpha-interferon therapy. J Hepatol 1992 ; 16 : 380-3.
23. Shindo M, Di Bisceglie AM, Biswas R, Mihalik K, Feinstone SM. Hepatitis C virus replication during acute infection in the chimpanzee. J Infect Dis 1992 ; 166 : 424-7.
24. Lanford RE, Notvall L, Chavez D, White R, Frenzel G, Simonsen C, Kim J. Analysis of hepatitis C virus capsid E1, and E2/NS1 proteins expressed in insect cells. Virology 1993 ; 197 : 225-35.
25. Ralston R, Thudium K, Berger K, Kuo C, Gervase B, Hall J, Selby M, Kuo G, Houghton M, Choo QL. Characterization of hepatitis C virus envelope glycoprotein complexes expressed by recombinant vaccinia viruses. Virology 1993 ; 67 : 6753-61.
26. Wang C, Sarnow P, Siddiqui A. Translation of human hepatitis C virus RNA in cultured cells is mediated by an internal ribosome-binding mechanism. J Virol 1993 ; 67 : 3338-44.
27. Higashi Y, Kakumu S, Yoshioka K, Watika T, Mizokami M, Ohba K, Ito Y, Ishikawa T, Takayanagi M, Nagai Y. Dynamics of genome change in the E2/NS1 region of hepatitis C virus in vivo. Virology 1993 ; 197 : 659-68.
28. Bukh J, Purcell RH, Miller RH. At least 12 genotypes of hepatitis C virus predicted by sequence analysis of the putative E1 gene of isolates collected worldwide. Proc Natl Acad Sci USA 1993 ; 90 : 8234-8.
29. Simmonds P, Holmes EC, Cha TA, Chan SW, McHomish F, Irvine B, Beall E, Yap PL, Kolberg J, Urdea MS. Classification of hepatitis C virus into six major genotypes and a series of subtypes by phylogenetic analysis of the NS-5 region. Journal of general virology 1993 ; 74 : 2391-9.
30. Kurosaki M, Enomoto N, Marumo F, Sato C. Rapid sequence variation of the hypervariable region of hepatitis C virus during the course of chronic infection. Hepatology 1993 ; 18 : 1293-9.
31. Cha T, Beall T, Irvine B, Kolberg J, Chien D, Kuo G. At least five related, but distinct, hepatitis C viral genotypes exist. Proc Natl Acad Sci USA 1992 ; 89 : 7144-8.
32. Chan S, McOmish F, Holmes E, Dow B, Peutherer J, Follett E. Analysis of a new hepa-

titis C virus type and its phylogenetic relationship to existing variants. J Gen Virol 1992 ; 73 : 1131-41.
33. Enomoto N, Takada A, Nakao T, Date T. There are two major types of hepatitis C virus in Japan. Biochem Biophys Res Commun 1990 ; 170 : 1021-5.
34. Takamizawa A, Mori C, Fuke I, *et al.* Structure and organization of the hepatitis C virus genome isolated from human carriers. J Virol 1991 ; 65 : 1105-13.
35. Okamoto H, Kurai K, Okada S-I, *et al.* Full-length sequence of a hepatitis C virus genome having poor homology to reported isolates : comparative study of four distinct genotypes. Virology 1992 ; 188 : 331-41.
36. Bukh J, Purcell R, Miller R. At least 12 genotypes of hepatitis C virus predicted by sequence analysis of the putative E1 gene of isolates collected worldwide. Proc Natl Acad Sci USA 1993 ; 90 : 8234-8.
37. Li J, Tong S, Vitvitski L, Lepot D, Trepo C. Two French genotypes of hepatitis C virus : homology of the predominant genotype with the prototype American strain. Gene 1991 ; 105 : 167-72.
38. Okamoto H, Kojima M, Okada S-I, *et al.* Genetic drift of hepatitis C virus during an 8.2-year infection in a chimpanzee : variability and stability. Virology 1992 ; 190 : 894-9.
39. Simmonds P, McOmish F, Yap P, *et al.* Sequence variability in the 5' non-coding region of hepatitis C virus : identification of a new virus type and restrictions on sequence diversity. J Gen Virol 1993 ; 74 : 661-8.
40. Nakao T, Enomoto N, Takada N, Takada A, Date T. Typing of hepatitis C virus genomes by restriction fragment length polymorphism. J Gen Virol 1991 ; 72 : 2105-12.
41. McOmish F, Chan S, Dow B, *et al.* Detection of three types of hepatitis C virus in blood donors : investigation of type-specific differences in serologic reactivity and rate of alanine aminotransferase abnormalities. Transfusion 1993 ; 33 : 7-13.
42. Okamoto H, Sugiyama Y, Okada S, *et al.* Typing hepatitis C virus by polymerase chain reaction with type-specific primers : application to clinical surveys and tracing infectious sources. J Gen Virol 1992 ; 73 : 673-9.
43. Okamoto H, Tokita H, Sakamoto M, *et al.* Characterization of the genomic sequence of type-V (or 3a) hepatitis C virus isolates and PCR primers for specific detection. J Gen Virol 1993 ; 74 : 2385-90.
44. Stuyver L, Rossay R, Wyseur A, *et al.* Typing of hepatitis C virus isolates and characterization of new subtypes using a line probe assay. J Gen Virol 1993 ; 74 : 1093-109.
45. Lai ME, Mazzoleni AP, Argiolu F, De Virgilis S, Balestrieri A, Purcell RH, Cao A, Farci P. Hepatitis C virus in multiple episodes of acute hepatitis in polytransfused thalassaemic children. Lancet 1994 ; 343 : 388-90.
46. Féray C, Gigou M, Samuel D, *et al.* Hepatitis C virus RNA and hepatitis B virus DNA in serum and liver of patients with fulminant hepatitis. Gastroenterology 1993 ; 104 : 549-55.
47. Weiner A, Geysen H, Christopherson C, *et al.* Evidence for immune selection of hepatitis C virus (HCV) putative envelope glycoprotein variants : potential role in chronic HCV infections. Proc Natl Acad Sci USA 1992 ; 89 : 3468-72.
48. Chemello L, Alberti A, Kenneth R, Simmonds P. Hepatitis C serotype and response to interferon therapy. N Engl J Med 1994 ; 330 : 143.
49. Kobayashi Y, Watanabe S, Konishi M, Yokoi M, Kakehashi R, Kaito M, Kondo M, Hayashi Y, Jomori T, Suzuki S. Quantitation and typing of serum hepatitis C virus RNA in patients with chronic hepatitis C treated with interferon-β. Hepatology 1993 ; 18 : 1319-25.
50. Yoshioka K, Kakumu S, Wakita T, *et al.* Detection of hepatitis C virus by polymerase chain reaction and response to interferon-alpha therapy : relationship to genotypes of hepatitis C virus. Hepatology 1992 ; 16 : 293-9.
51. Brouwer J, Nevens F, Kleter G, *et al.* Which hepatitis C patient will benefit from interferon ? Multivariate analysis of 350 patients treated in a Benelux mulicentre study. J Hepatol 1993 ; 18, Suppl 1 : S10.
52. Takada N, Takase S, Takada A, Date T. Differences in the hepatitis C virus genotypes in different countries. J Hepatol 1993 ; 17 : 277-83.

53. Pozzato G, Moretti M, Franzin F, *et al.* Severity of liver disease with different hepatitis C viral clones. Lancet 1991 ; 338 : 509 (Letter).
54. Pozzato G, Moretti M, Franzin F, *et al.* The presence of « Japanese type » of NS4 region is associated to more severe liver disease. J. Hepatol. 1992 ; 16 : S3.
55. Kato N, Sekiya H, Ootsuyama Y, *et al.* Humoral Immune response to hypervariable region 1 of the putative envelope glycoprotein (gp70) of hepatitis C virus. J Virol 1993 ; 67 : 3923-30.
56. Okada SI, Akahane Y, Suzuki H, Okamoto H, Mishiro S. The degree of variability in the amino terminal region of the E2/NS1 protein of hepatitis C virus correlates with responsiveness to interferon therapy in viremic patients. Hepatology 1992 ; 16 : 619-24.
57. Sherman K, O'Brien J, Gutierrez A, *et al.* Quantitative evaluation of hepatitis C virus RNA in patients with concurrent human immunodeficiency virus infections. J Clin Microbiol 1993 ; 31 : 2679-82.
58. Shimizu YK, Hijikata M, Iwamoto A, Alter HJ, Purcell RH, Yoshikura H. Neutralizing antibodies against hepatitis C virus ande the emergence of neutralization escape mutant virus. Journal of virology 1994 ; 68 : 1494-500.
59. Shimizu Y, Purcell RH, Yoshikura H. Correlation between the infectivity of hepatitis C virus in vivo and its infectivity *in vitro*. Proc Natl Acad 1993 ; 90 : 6037-41.
60. Bottarelli P, Brunetto MR, Minutello MA, Calvo P, Unutmaz D, Weiner AJ, Choo QL, Shuster JR, Kuo G, Bonino F, Houghton M, Abrignani S. T-Lymphocyte response to hepatitis C virus in different clinical course of infection. Gastroenterology 1993 ; 104 : 580-7.
61. Knodell R, Ishak K, Black W, *et al.* Formulation and application of a numerical scoring system for assessing histological activity in asymptomatic chronic active hepatitis. Hepatology 1981 ; 1 : 431-5.
62. Chomczynski P, Sacchi N. Single-step method of RNA isolation by acid guanidium thiocyanate-phenol-chloroform extraction. Analyt Biochem 1987 ; 162 : 156-9.
63. Kwok S, Higushi R. Avoiding false positive results with PCR. Nature 1989 ; 339 : 237-8.

2

Significance of indeterminate second generation RIBA and resolution by third generation RIBA

J.-M. PAWLOTSKY

*Department of Bacteriology and Virology
Hôpital Henri-Mondor, Université Paris-XII, 94010 Créteil, France.*

The diagnosis of hepatitis C virus (HCV) infections is primarily based on the specific detection of anti-HCV antibodies by enzyme immunoassays. These assays evidence antibodies directed to both structural and non structural viral antigens. They are easy to perform, rather cheap and allow testing of large series of samples because they are automated in most cases. However, they may lead to false positive results due to non specific binding of serum immunoglobulins onto antigen-coated microwells or beads. For this reason, validation of enzyme immunoassay results appears to be necessary by means of more specific strip immunoblot assays (SIA) [1-11]. The most widely used SIA worldwide is the second generation recombinant immunoblot assay (RIBA HCV 2.0 SIA or RIBA2.0) developed by Chiron Corporation (Emeryville CA, USA) and commercialized by Ortho Diagnostic Systems (Raritan NJ, USA). RIBA2.0 has been shown to be both more sensitive and more specific than the first generation RIBA [3, 4, 7, 8, 10, 12]. According to the manufacturer's instructions, RIBA 2.0 may give three kinds of patterns : positive, negative, or indeterminate [2]. Indeterminate results are difficult to interpret in terms of viral disease, so that the development of new SIAs, designed to avoid such patterns appears to be mandatory. Third generation RIBA (RIBA HCV 3.0 SIA or RIBA3.0) was recently developed and begins to be routinely used in France and in some European countries.

Principles and interpretation of the RIBA HCV SIA

Principles of the tests

RIBA HCV SIA have been designed for the validation of positive results of second or third generation enzyme-linked immunosorbent assays (ELISA2.0 and ELISA3.0, Ortho Diagnostic Systems). RIBA HCV SIA are nitrocellulose-based tests which qualitatively detect antibodies to HCV-encoded antigens in serum and plasma. In the RIBA2.0, four HCV recombinant proteins are immobilized as individual bands on nitrocellulose strips, the same matrix as is used in Western blots. These four recombinant proteins are derived from the nucleocapsid (structural antigen c22-3) and the NS3-NS4 regions of the HCV genome (non structural antigens 5.1.1, c100-3, c33c). During the incubation of the strips with serum or plasma specimens or the appropriate controls, antibodies to HCV, if present, react with the corresponding recombinant antigen bands on the nitrocellulose strips. After the removal of non specific antibodies by aspiration and washing, the strips are then reacted with goat anti-human IgG conjugated with horseradish peroxydase. Following incubation, decantation and washing to remove excess conjugate, a solution containing peroxyde and 4-chloro-1-naphtol is added. Band patterns develop on each strip. The intensity of the blue-black colored band is proportional to the amount of specific antibody bound to each of the HCV recombinant antigens on the strips. After the development of color on the strips, the reaction is stopped by decantation and washing. The reactivity of specimens towards each recombinant antigen is determined by visually comparing the intensity of the individual band with that of the low and high IgG internal control bands included on each strip.

The recently developed RIBA3.0 differs from RIBA2.0 as follows : *a)* recombinant 5.1.1 and c100-3 proteins were replaced by a mixture of both 5.1.1 and c100 synthetic peptides ; *b)* a conformationally modified recombinant c33c protein was added to the initial c33c ; *c)* recombinant c22-3 protein was replaced by a four-epitope c22 synthetic peptide ; these modifications, together with changes in the technical procedure improving the specificity of the assay, allowed to significantly increase the amount of epitopes present on the strips ; *d)* furthermore, a recombinant NS5 protein was added. In spite of these modifications, the principle and the interpretation of the test are similar to those of RIBA2.0.

Interpretation of RIBA HCV SIA

According to the manufacturer's instructions, the patterns of the strips have to be interpreted by comparing the antigen band intensity to the level I and level II strip controls as follows (Table I)

Table I.

Antigen band response	Rating
no visible band	−
visible band : intensity less than level I control	+/−
visible band : intensity equal to level I control	1+
visible band : intensity greater than level I and less than level II	2+
visible band : intensity equal to level II control	3+
visible band : intensity greater than level II control	4+

A response of 1+ or greater indicates sample reactivity to a given antigen, whereas visible reactivity scored +/- is considered to be non reactive to a given antigen. The results must therefore be interpreted as follows :
— no bands of 1+ or greater reactivity present : negative,
— 1+ or greater reactivity to any two HCV recombinant antigens : positive,
— only one band of 1+ or greater reactivity present, whereas pattern does not meet criteria for positive : indeterminate.

Indeterminate RIBA2.0 in blood donors

Results of RIBA2.0 in blood donors with repeatedly reactive ELISA2.0

The prevalences of the different RIBA2.0 patterns observed in series of blood donors with repeatedly reactive ELISA2.0 are presented on the Table II.

From these results, it appears that almost half of the blood donors with repeatedly reactive ELISA2.0 can be definitely considered negative for the presence of anti-HCV antibodies according to the result of RIBA2.0. However, about one third of these donors is found to have an indeterminate pattern, raising the problem of the significance of such pattern.

Table II.

	Number of ELISA2.0 (+) blood donors	RIBA2.0 Positive	RIBA2.0 Indeterminate	RIBA2.0 Negative
Bresters et al. [13]	1105	17 %	38 %	45 %
Boudart et al. [14]	126	15 %	33 %	52 %
El Ghouzzi et al. [15]	717	36 %	23 %	41 %
Follett et al. [16]	169	29 %	22 %	49 %
Sayers and Gretch [17]	151	52 %	34 %	14 %

Significance of the different RIBA2.0 patterns observed in blood donors with repeatedly reactive ELISA2.0

The only direct test evidencing viral replication, i.e., active viral infection, is the detection of HCV RNA by the polymerase chain reaction (PCR) [18, 19]. Few data are available on the significance, in terms of viral replication, of the different RIBA2.0 patterns observed in blood donors with repeatedly reactive ELISA2.0. The results of three recent studies, reporting the prevalences of positive PCR according to RIBA2.0 pattern in blood donors, are presented in the following Table III.

Table III.

	RIBA2.0 positive	% of positive PCR RIBA2.0 negative	RIBA2.0 indeterminate
Bresters et al. [13]	75 %	0 %	2 %
Sayers and Gretch [17]	73 %	0 %	14 %
Follett et al. [20]	84 %	0 %	5 %

Therefore, the interpretation of RIBA2.0 as indeterminate appears unsatisfactory in blood donors, because most of them have no viral replication and should be considered negative, whereas some of them are found to have serum HCV RNA by PCR and should be considered positive. Thus, these results emphasize the need for more discriminative tests.

Value of RIBA3.0 in blood donors with indeterminate RIBA2.0

In a study performed in the Ruchill Hospital of Glasgow (UK), 5 % of 130 blood donors with indeterminate RIBA2.0 were found to have serum HCV RNA by PCR (Follett). All these 130 sera were tested by RIBA3.0. Among those with negative PCR, 61 % became negative with this test, 14 % became positive and 25 % remained indeterminate. Among those with positive PCR, none became negative, 61 % became positive and 39 % remained indeterminate. This result is due to a significant improvement in the predictive value of RIBA3.0 compared to RIBA2.0 with regard to viral replication in blood donors. This point is illustrated on the Table IV where the results of indeterminate RIBA2.0 resolution by RIBA3.0 are presented, according to the initial indeterminate RIBA2.0 pattern (A. Polito, personal communication).

Table IV.

RIBA2.0 indeterminate pattern	Number of samples tested	% resolved by RIBA3.0	% indeterminate RIBA3.0
c100-3	54	89 % (0 % pos/89 % neg)	11 %
c33c	387	70 % (20 % pos/50 % neg)	30 %
c22-3	107	80 % (34 % pos/46 % neg)	20 %

In summary, RIBA3.0 may resolve most cases of indeterminate RIBA2.0 in blood donors with repeatedly reactive ELISA2.0. However, rare samples may remain RIBA3.0 indeterminate, some of which may be HCV RNA positive by PCR.

Indeterminate RIBA2.0 in patients detected ELISA2.0 positive in virology laboratories

The discovery of an indeterminate RIBA2.0 pattern in a laboratory of virology is a different setting, because the samples routinely tested come from patients, who usually have symptoms of liver disease and/or risk factors for HCV infection justifying the search for anti-HCV antibodies.

Results of RIBA2.0 in patients detected ELISA2.0 positive in virology laboratories

In our hospital laboratory, 5,872 ELISA2.0s were performed between July 1991 and July 1992. Among them, 1,306 were found positive, leading to validation by RIBA2.0. Among these 1,306 sera, 922 (71 %) were RIBA2.0 positive, 177 (13 %) were RIBA2.0 negative and 207 (16 %) were RIBA2.0 indeterminate. When detected in virology laboratories, RIBA2.0 indeterminate patterns are characterized in most cases by the presence of an isolated c22-3 or c33c band on the strip, whereas c100-3 and 5.1.1 profiles are very rare, as shown on the Table V

Table V.

	Indeterminate RIBA2.0 pattern			
	c22-3	c33c	c100-3	5.1.1
Pawlotsky et al. [21] (n = 207)	73 %	23 %	4 %	0 %
Lunel et al. [22] (n = 143)	69 %	27 %	4 %	0 %
Buffet et al. [23] (n = 57)	81 %	16 %	3 %	0 %

Significance of indeterminate RIBA2.0 patterns in patients tested in virology laboratories

Indeterminate RIBA2.0 profiles detected in laboratories of virology seem to be associated with immunosuppression in a large number of patients. Indeed, this was the case in 51 % of the 143 patients of Lunel et al.'s series, including 53 % of c22-3 indeterminate and 56 % of c33c indeterminate subjects [21]. In the series of Buffet et al., immunosuppression was found in 65 % of the patients with indeterminate RIBA2.0 [23]. We studied 60 patients with an indeterminate RIBA2.0 profile characterized by the presence of a highly positive (3+ or 4+) c22-3 band on the strip [21]. Forty-two of them (70 %) were immunocompromised. This prevalence was significantly higher than that in patients with positive RIBA2.0 (35 %, $p < 0.001$). This result could be explained by impaired production of anti-HCV antibodies in immunocompromised patients, so that the amount of some of these antibodies could be lower than the cutoff of the assay. Severe immunosuppression could even be responsible for falsely negative RIBA patterns. However, it is noteworthy that some patients without any cause of immunosuppression can be found to have indeterminate RIBA2.0. The reason why these patients could produce lower amounts of anti-HCV antibodies is still unclear.

In most series from virology laboratories, a large proportion of the patients with indeterminate RIBA2.0 is found to have risk factors for HCV infection and raised serum ALT (83 % and 77 % in our series, respectively [21]). In the same way, most of these patients are found to be HCV RNA positive by PCR, as suggested by the following results (Table VI).

Table VI.

	Positive PCR
Pawlotsky et al. [21] : highly positive c22-3 indeterminate RIBA2.0	83 %
immunocompromised patients (n = 42)	88 %
non immunocompromised patients (n = 18)	72 %
patients with raised ALT (n = 46)	87 %
patients with repeatedly normal ALT (n = 14)	71 %
Lunel et al. [22] : c22-3 and c33c indeterminate RIBA2.0	
immunocompromised patients (n = 20)	85 %
non immunocompromised patients (n = 16)	44 %
Martinot-Peignoux et al. [24] : all patterns of indeterminate RIBA2.0	47 %

Since indeterminate RIBA2.0 profiles are associated in most cases with HCV replication evidenced by positive PCR, the term « indeterminate » appears to be unsatisfactory. This fact emphasizes the need for a more discriminative test.

Value of RIBA3.0 in patients with indeterminate RIBA2.0 detected in virology laboratories

Preliminary data obtained from French laboratories, where RIBA3.0 has now been routinely used for several months, show that most cases of indeterminate RIBA2.0 may be resolved by RIBA3.0. The Table VII presents the prevalences of positive RIBA3.0 according to indeterminate RIBA2.0 pattern.

Table VII.

	Overall	Indeterminate RIBA2.0 profile			
		c22-3	c33c	c100-3	5.1.1
Pawlotsky et al. [21]	NP	85 % (n = 60)	NP	NP	NP
Lunel et al. [22]	NP	33 % (n = 98)	59 % (n = 39)	NP	NP
Buffet et al. [23]	58 % (n = 57)	59 % (n = 46)	66 % (n = 9)	0 % (n = 2)	NP
Martinot-Peignoux et al. [24]	57 % (n = 51)	NP	NP	NP	NP

NP = not performed

These results suggest that RIBA3.0 is found positive in about 60 % of the patients having indeterminate RIBA2.0, the majority of whose is represented by c22-3 and c33c indeterminate patterns. The resolution of indeterminate RIBA2.0 by RIBA3.0 was due in most cases to a significant improvement in the detection of anti-c100, anti-c33c and anti-c22 antibodies. Indeed, in our series of c22-3 indeterminate RIBA2.0, 94 % of the patients had positive c33c and 67 % had positive c100 [21]. The addition of a NS5 antigen on the strip did not appear to have great value in these series, because all the patients who had anti-NS5 antibodies also had at least one other antibody present, so that resolution was never achieved by NS5 alone [21, 23]. However, a few high risk RIBA2.0 indeterminates were confirmed positive by RIBA3.0 because of addition reactivity to NS5 only in another series (A. Polito, personal communication).

It is of interest to note that some patients with indeterminate RIBA2.0 were found to be either RIBA3.0 negative or RIBA3.0 indeterminate. In this last case, they were characterized by the presence of the same band in RIBA3.0 as in RIBA2.0. These results are presented on the Table VIII.

From these results, it can be concluded that, although RIBA3.0 allows to resolve the majority of indeterminate RIBA2.0 patterns, indeterminate RIBA3.0 profiles may still be observed. In our series, 6 among the 9 patients who remained RIBA3.0 indeterminate had HCV RNA detected by PCR : these 6 patients had raised serum alanine aminotransferase activity and severe immunosuppression [21]. PCR was also positive in 4 among the 11 patients with indeterminate RIBA3.0

reported by Martinot-Peignoux et al. [24] and 15 among the 20 patients tested by Buffet et al. [23].

Table VIII.

	Indeterminate RIBA2.0 pattern	RIBA3.0 pattern	
		Negative	Indeterminate
Pawlotsky et al. [21]	highly positive c22-3 (n = 60)	0 %	15 %
Lunel et al. [22]	c33c (n = 39)	2 %	38 %
	c22-3 (n = 98)	1 %	66 %
Buffet et al. [23]	c100-3 (n = 2)	100 %	0 %
	c33c (n = 46)	0 %	41 %
	c22-3 (n = 9)	0 %	33 %
Martinot-Peignoux et al. [24]	Overall (n = 51)	22 %	22 %

Significance of indeterminate RIBA3.0

In a recent work performed by the Groupe d'Études Moléculaires des Hépatites (GEMHEP), 89 observations of indeterminate RIBA3.0 patterns from 10 French centers (7 laboratories of virology and 3 blood centers) were studied [25]. All patterns of indeterminate RIBA3.0 were observed, including c22 (75 %), c33c (16 %), c100 (6 %) and NS5 (3 %). HCV RNA was found positive by PCR in 61 % of c22 indeterminate, 57 % of c33c indeterminate and 60 % of c100 indeterminate RIBA3.0s. It is of interest to note that 63 % of these subjects were immunocompromized, suggesting that, although the sensitivity of RIBA3.0 has been significantly improved compared to RIBA2.0, some patients may have deeply impaired production of antibodies that could be present at levels lower than the cutoff of RIBA3.0. These results were confirmed by preliminary data from our laboratory (manuscript in preparation). We studied 50 consecutive indeterminate RIBA3.0 patterns and showed that these patterns could be characterized by the presence of any of the four bands. Moreover, HCV RNA was detected by PCR in 44 % of them, suggesting that the term « indeterminate » does not account for the actual replicative state of the virus in these patients.

In conclusion, indeterminate second generation RIBA profiles are frequently observed in low risk blood donors with repeatedly positive

ELISA2.0 as well as in patients tested in laboratories of virology because of risk factor for HCV infection and/or symptoms of liver disease. The recently developed third generation RIBA allows to resolve most of these diagnostic problems. However, indeterminate third generation RIBA profiles may still be observed. In this case, detection of HCV RNA by PCR appears to be mandatory to determine whether or not HCV replication is present. These results suggest that further improvement in the sensitivity and the specificity of the tests used for the detection of anti-HCV antibodies is needed.

References

1. Van Der Poel CL, Reesink HW, Lelie PN, et al. Anti-HCV and transaminase testing of blood donors. Lancet 1990 ; 336 : 187-8.
2. Van Der Poel CL, Cuypers HTM, Reesink HW, et al. Confirmation of hepatitis C virus infection by new four-antigen recombinant immunoblot assay. Lancet 1991 ; 337 : 317-9.
3. Marcellin P, Martinot-Peignoux M, Boyer N, et al. Second generation RIBA test in diagnosis of chronic hepatitis C. Lancet 1991 ; 337 : 552.
4. Leon A, Canton R, Elia M, Mateos M. Second generation RIBA to confirm diagnosis of HCV infection. Lancet 1991 ; 337 : 912.
5. Gretch D, Lee W, Corey L. Use of aminotransferase, hepatitis C antibody, and hepatitis C polymerase chain reaction RNA assays to establish the diagnosis of hepatitis C virus infection in a diagnostic virology laboratory. J Clin Microbiol 1992 ; 30 : 2145-9.
6. Da Silva Cardoso M, Jochem H, Hesse R, Epple S, Koerner K, Kubanek B. Evaluating recombinant protein immunoblot assay and polymerase chain reaction for diagnosis of non-A, non-B hepatitis. J Infect Dis 1992 ; 166 : 450-1.
7. Alter HJ. New kit on the block : evaluation of second generation assays for detection of antibody to hepatitis C virus. Hepatology 1992 ; 15 : 350-3.
8. Nakatsuji Y, Matsumoto A, Tanaka E, Ogata H, Kiyosawa K. Detection of chronic hepatitis C virus infection by four diagnostic systems : first generation and second generation enzyme-linked immunosorbent assay, second generation recombinant immunoblot assay and nested polymerase chain reaction analysis. Hepatology 1992 ; 16 : 300-5.
9. Frost EH. Investigation of sera reactive to hepatitis C virus by second generation enzyme immunoassay. J Clin Microbiol 1993 ; 31 : 163-4.
10. Yuki N, Hayashi N, Hagiwara H, et al. Serodiagnosis of chronic hepatitis C in Japan by second generation recombinant immunoblot assay. J Hepatol 1993 ; 17 : 170-4.
11. Shev S, Foberg U, Fryden A, et al. Second generation hepatitis C ELISA antibody tests confirmed by the four-antigen recombinant immunoblot assay correlate well with hepatitis C viraemia and chronic liver disease in Swedish blood donors. Vox Sang 1993 ; 65 : 32-7.
12. Farci P, London WT, Wong DC, et al. The natural history of infection with hepatitis C virus (HCV) in chimpanzees : comparison of serologic responses measured with first and second generation assays and relationship to HCV viraemia. J Infect Dis 1992 ; 165 : 1006-11.
13. Bresters D, Zaaijer HL, Cuypers HTM, et al. Recombinant immunoblot assay reaction patterns and hepatitis C virus RNA in blood donors and non-A, non-B hepatitis patients. Transfusion 1993 ; 33 : 634-8.
14. Boudart D, Lucas JC, Adjou C, Muller JY. HCV confirmatory testing of blood donors. Lancet 1992 ; 339 : 372.
15. El Ghouzzi MH, N'Dalla J, Vuittenez MC, Desaint C, Nubel L. Unpublished data.

16. Follett EAC, Dow BC, Mc Omish F, *et al.* HCV confirmatory testing of blood donors. Lancet 1991 ; 338 : 1024.
17. Sayers MH, Gretch DR. Recombinant immunoblot and polymerase chain reaction testing in volunteer whole blood donors screened by a multiantigen assay for hepatitis C virus antibodies. Transfusion 1993 ; 33 : 809-13.
18. Weiner AJ, Kuo G, Bradley DW, *et al.* Detection of hepatitis C viral sequences in non-A, non-B hepatitis. Lancet 1990 ; 335 : 1-3.
19. Garson JA, Tedder RS, Briggs M, *et al.* Detection of hepatitis C viral sequences in blood donations by « nested » polymerase chain reaction and prediction of infectivity. Lancet 1990 ; 335 : 1419-22.
20. Follett EAC. unpublished data.
21. Pawlotsky JM, Fleury A, Choukroun V, *et al.* Significance of highly positive c22-3 « indeterminate » second generation hepatitis C virus (HCV) recombinant immunoblot assay (RIBA) and resolution by third generation HCV RIBA. J Clin Microbiol 1994 ; 32 : 1357-9.
22. Lunel F, Perrin M, Frangeul L, Aumont P, Opolon P, Huraux JM. Sensitivity of third generation Ortho HCV ELISA and RIBA in 143 patients with indeterminate second generation RIBA. In : Abstract Book of the Fourth International Symposium on HCV. Ortho Diagnostic Systems and Chiron Corporation, eds. Tokyo, Japan, 1993 : 72.
23. Buffet C, Charnaux N, Laurent-Puig P, *et al.* Enhanced detection of antibodies to hepatitis C virus by use of a third generation recombinant immunoblot assay. J Med Virol 1994 ; in press.
24. Martinot-Peignoux M, Gabriel F, Branger M, *et al.* Detection of antibodies to hepatitis C virus (HCV) by second and third generation anti-HCV testing with comparison to polymerase chain reaction. Manuscript submitted.
25. Lamoril J, Lunel F, Laurent-Puig P, *et al.* Indeterminate third generation recombinant immunoblot assay in hepatitis C virus infections. J Hepatol 1994 ; in press.

3
Role of liver disease and hepatitis C virus infection in the pathogenesis of mixed cryoglobulinemia

L. MUSSET[1], F. LUNEL[2]

[1] Service d'Immunochimie ;
[2] Service de Bactério-virologie,
Groupe Hospitalier Pitié-Salpêtrière,
43-47, boulevard de l'Hôpital, 75651 Paris Cedex 13, France.

Cryoglobulins (CG) represent a particular group of serum proteins which share the property of precipitation at temperatures below 37 °C. Conventionally, CG are classified according to their immunoglobulins (Ig) composition : monoclonal Ig alone (type I), both monoclonal and polyclonal Ig (type II) or polyclonal Ig (type III) [1]. An enrichment of IgM with rheumatoid factor (RF) activity is consistently observed in mixed CG (type II and III), as well as an enrichment of IgG1 and IgG3 subclasses suggesting that cryoprecipitation of Ig are specific antigen-antibody complexes, rather than a merely non-specific precipitation of cold-insoluble proteins [2, 3]. Mixed cryoglobulinemias are a systemic disorder characterized by cutaneous vasculitis and visceral complications, mainly renal, neurologic and liver [1, 4]. As a syndrome, cryoglobulinemia is associated with a wide variety of lymphoproliferative diseases, acute or chronic infections, and auto-immune diseases. If no primary disorder is found, mixed CG are classified as « essential » mixed cryoglobulinemia (EMC) [5, 6].

The reports about the association between cryoglobulinemia and liver involvement are well documented [7-10], but still raise several conflicting hypothesis concerning the pathogenesis of mixed CG and the underlying liver disorder. Recently, it has been recognized that viral infection, in particular the hepatitis C, appear to be involved in the pathogenesis of the main essential form of cryoglobulinemia [11-23]. The purpose of this review is to focus on the main clinical and biological findings about this association of mixed CG with hepatitis C virus infection (HCV). On this point of view, HCV infection is of particular interest to help to delineating the immunopathological effects of cryoglobulinemias and to explain the clinical and biological features (in particular immunological abnormalities) encountered in acute or chronic liver diseases.

Essential mixed cryoglobulinemia and liver diseases

The association between liver disease and cryoglobulinemia was first recognized many years ago [24, 25], but its pathophysiological significance is still poorly understood. Initialy, the term « essential » mixed CG (first described by Meltzer & Franklin in 1966) [5] has been used to designate patients with a specific syndrome consisting of purpura, weakness and arthralgias. However, these authors observed clinical and biological liver abnormalities in 9 out of 26 patients (35 %) with EMC. Several studies have since confirmed the frequency of mixed cryoglobulinemia in various liver diseases (both acute and chronic), and vice versa [9, 27]. There is marked controversy surrounding the link between EMC and liver diseases. Several authors consider that liver disease, regardless of the etiology, is one of the main causes of mixed cryoglobulinemia, while others view the EMC described by Meltzer & Franklin as a form of necrotizing vasculitis, the etiologic agent of which also causes liver lesions [4, 8, 9, 26, 27].

In 1977, Levo et al. [28] suggested the involvement of hepatitis B virus (HBV) in the pathogenesis of EMC. They effectively diagnosed liver disease in 26 out of 30 patients (86 %) with EMC, and detected HBV markers (HBs antigen and/or anti-HBs antibody) in 15 out of 25 sera (60 %) and 14 out of 19 cryoprecipitates (74 %). Viral particles were also observed in four cryoprecipitates examined under the electron microscope. These authors proposed that the term « EMC » should be replaced in most of the cases by « mixed CG secondary to infection by HBV or another unidentified virus ». In this hypothesis, mixed cryoglobulinemia is considered as one of the extra-hepatic manifestations of viral B hepatitis. However, these observations have not been confirmed by other authors, including ourselves [29-31]. This discrepancy could at least partly be due to a patient selection bias or differences in the definition of EMC. In addition, interference by IgM with RF activity in the tests used to detect specific antibodies or antigens was not ruled out in several studies, including that of Levo et al. [28]. Yet several authors have shown that when specific antibody activity is detected, it is usually present in the IgG fraction of the cryoprecipitate rather than the IgM fraction [21, 34].

Mixed cryoglobulinemia and hepatitis C virus infection

Role of the hepatitis C virus

Recent progress in molecular biology has made it possible to diagnose viral C hepatitis. Several authors have observed that some cases of EMC were in fact active viral C hepatitis. The association between cryoglobulinemia and HCV is now well documented. A high frequency of HCV markers (anti-HCV antibodies and/or HCV-RNA) has been reported in patients'sera with mixed CG (86 % in the report by Ferri et al. [12], 48 % in the report by Casato et al. [14] and 42 % in the report by Dammacco et al. [18]). Our own studies of two large series of patients have shown a prevalence of cryoglobulinemia of 54.3 % in patients infected by HCV [31], and a prevalence of HCV infection of 52 % in patients with EMC [19, 32]. However, is this sufficient to consider that HCV is the principal etiological agent in mixed cryoglobulinemia ?

Mixed CG has occasionally been observed in patients with viral A hepatitis [33]. The high prevalence of markers of HBV infection reported by Levo et al. [28] was not confirmed in later studies [29, 30], including those by our group in which 15 % of patients with viral B hepatitis had cryoglobulinemia [31]. Among the other viral infections studied so far (cytomegalovirus, Epstein Barr virus and herpes viruses) [34, 35], none has been as strongly linked to cryoglobulinemia as HCV. However, several problems have arisen since the first studies reported in 1991. Indeed, most of these studies involved small numbers of cases or particular recruitment ; this was especially the case of Italian studies, in which the geographic distribution of HCV and cryoglobulinemias was similar. In addition, the use of first-generation ELISA tests could have led to false-positive results, particularly with hypergammaglobulinemic sera and sera containing RF. Several studies, including our own, have since ruled out false-positive results and recruitment bias, by means of second-generation ELISA and second or third-generation recombinant immunoblot assay (RIBA) tests and the detection of HCV-RNA by the polymerase chain reaction (PCR).

The hypothetic role of HCV in the pathogenesis of cryoglobulinemia has been recently reinforced by the detection of HCV-RNA in cryoprecipitates, at higher concentrations that in the corresponding sera and serum supernatants (Table I) [21, 31, 36]. We have also detected specific anti-HCV antibody activity, as well as viral core proteins in the cryoprecipitate. This points to the presence of encapsidated RNA and virion particles in the cryoprecipitate. These observations together with reduction or elimination of CG during interferon therapy reported in the literature [37-39] and in our experience [31] are also indirect arguments favoring the role of HCV in the onset of mixed CG.

Table I. Concentration of HCV RNA (Eq/ml $\times$ 10^5) measured using branched DNA (Quantiplex, Chiron Corporation, Emeryville, CA) in supernatant, serum, and cryoprecipiate of 5 patients with hepatitis C and cryoglobulinemia.

Patients N°	Supernatant	Serum	Cryoprecipitate
1	15.62	15.53	> 560
2	25.8	51.3	117
3	10.45	35.3	68.2
4	25	25	28
5	7.7	30	99

CG could be composed of specific antigen (HCV)-antibody complexes and IgM with RF activity, which would trap and eliminate the virus *in vivo*. In fact, the antigens involved in the formation of CG are rarely identified. Auto- and hetero-antigens have often been incriminated, but their nature and role have rarely been proven. There is still no proof of a direct role of the virus (or viral antigens) in the observed cryoprecipitates, while electron microscopic detection of viral particles has been fruitless.

Role of liver disease

Mixed CG (generally type III and low-level) has often been associated to acute or chronic liver disease. Altered hepatic clearance may play an important role in the onset or persistence of cryoglobulinemia [9, 10, 26]. If so, is liver damage a necessary step in the development of CG ?

In our study of HCV-infected patients [31], cryoglobulinemia appeared to be related to the presence of cirrhosis and the time since onset of the liver disease. It is very difficult to determine which factor is most directly involved. Indeed, although the degree of liver damage, assessed by means of the Knodell score [40] (or separate analysis of the fibrosis and inflammation scores) does not differ according to the presence or absence of cryoglobulinemia (Table II); the latter is nonetheless significantly more frequent in cirrhotic than in noncirrhotic patients (38 out of 55 (69 %) vs 31 out of 72 (43 %), $p < 0.01$). As cirrhosis is generally of insidious onset, the vast majority of these patients have a longer history of hepatitis and more severe liver damage. However, in a large number of cases, liver damage alone cannot account for cryoglobulinemia. Indeed, CG is diagnosed in 31 out of 72 (43 %) of noncirrhotic patients infected by HCV. In addition, the level of cryoglobulinemia and the frequency of clinical manifestations possibly related to it (cutaneous and/or vasomotor involvement, peripheral neuropathy, joint involvement, and renal involvement) are not different in cirrhotic and noncirrhotic patients (0.2 ± 0.3 vs 0.2 ± 0.3 g/L and 28 % vs 22 % respectively).

Table II. Main epidemiological and histological features in 127 patients with chronic hepatitis C with or without cyroglobulinemia (CG) (according to Lunel et al. [31].)

	Chronic hepatitis C		p
	With CG (n = 69)	Without CG (n = 58)	
Age (yrs)	52.8 ± 14	48.6 ± 16	NS
Sex ratio % (M/F)	45	59	NS
Duration of liver disease (yrs)	9.8 ± 10.6	5.3 ± 4.3	< 0.01
Knodell score	8.8 ± 2.3	8.1 ± 2.6	NS
Fibrosis score	2.6 ± 1.3	2 ± 1.2	NS
Cirrhosis (%)	55	29	< 0.01

NS, not significant

At the histological study in our experience, there was no significant difference in the frequency of lymphoid follicles between patients with and without cryoglobulinemia, ruling out an intrahepatic origin. Among HCV-infected patients, CG level was higher in patients with type II CG than those with type III CG, the detection of RF was also more frequent and the liver disease duration was longer (Table III) regardless of whether or not they have cirrhosis [31]. There is frequently an increase in the three classes of Ig. In the case of IgG, it

Table III. Main clinical and biological features of 69 patients with chronic hepatitis C and type II or type III cryoglobulinemia.

	Mixed cryoglobulinemia		p
	Type II (n = 22)	Type III (n = 47)	
Duration of liver disease (yrs)	14.2 ± 13.7	7.6 ± 7.7	< 0.01
Cryoglobulinemia (g/L)	0.38 ± 0.49	0.14 ± 0.11	< 0.01
Rheumatoid factor (%)	55	43	NS
Clinical feaures related to cryoglobulinemia*	6/22 (27 %)	12/47 (25 %)	NS
Knodell score	8.5 ± 3	8.7 ± 2.5	NS
Cirrhosis (%)	55	60	NS

NS, not significant
* Cutaneous and/or vasomotor signs, vasculitis, peripheral neuropathy, arthritis/arthralgias, renal involvement.

involves a selective and exclusive increase in IgG1, even in patients with moderate liver damage [41]. Prolonged antigenic stimulation, especially by protein antigens (viral or nonviral) may account for these observations. Another possible explanation for these cases of CG is an antigenic cross-reaction between HCV and the liver, particularly the diseased liver, or between HCV and an antigen encoded by the host genome, since some HCV-infected patients with mixed CG have no detectable liver damage [42]. In these two hypotheses, HCV infection eventually leads to the production of an auto-antibody recognizing both antigens.

In previous reports by Zarski et al. [9], Garcia-Bragado et al. [27] as well as in our experience [31] the prevalence of cryoglobulinemia varies greatly according to the type of disease. It was higher in alcoholics, and autoimmune liver disease (primary biliary cirrhosis and autoimmune hepatitis) than in other type of liver diseases. However, in patients with chronic hepatitis or cirrhosis unrelated to HCV, we reported that the prevalence of cryoglobulinemia is lower than in viral C hepatitis, even when liver damage is severe and cirrhosis is present [31]. Contrary to infection by HCV, the presence of cryoglobulinemia does not seem to be related to the duration of liver disease in these cases.

Taken together, these observations confirm the importance of HCV in the pathophysiology of mixed CG, but their development is difficult to dissociate from the nature and severity of liver damage. The pathogenesis of cryoglobulinemia in patients with liver diseases is no doubt multifactorial. The role of cirrhosis and/or the time since onset of the liver disease are determining factors, but several recent studies also reveal a special role of HCV (or possibly a particular HCV genotype) relative to other hepatotropic viruses. One plausible pathogenic hypothesis involves the immune reponse to a viral antigen or an auto-antigen.

References

1. Brouet JC, Clauvel JP, Danon F, Klein M, Seligmann M. Biologic and clinical significance of cryoglobulins. A report of 86 cases. Am J Med 1974 ; 57 : 775-88.
2. Renversez JC, Roussel S, Valle MJ, Lambert PH. Human type II mixed cryoglobulins as a model of idiotypic interactions. In : Ponticelli C, Minetti L, D'Amico G (eds) Antiglobulins, cryoglobulins and glomerulonephritis. Martinus Nijhoff, Dordrecht Boston Lancaster, 1986 ; 147-60.
3. Musset L, Duarte F, Gaillard O, Thi Huong Du L, Bilala J. Galli J, Preud'homme JL. Immunochemical characterization of monoclonal IgG containing mixed cryoglobulins. Clin Immunol Immunopathol 1994 ; 70 : 166-70.
4. Gorevic PD, Kassab HJ, Levo Y, Konh R, Meltzer M, Prose P, Franklin EC. Mixed cryoglobulinemia : clinical aspects and long term follow up of 40 patients. Am J Med 1980 ; 69 : 287-308.
5. Meltzer M, Franklin EC. Cryoglobulinemia — a study of 29 patients. Am J Med 1966 ; 40 : 828-36.
6. Meltzer M, Franklin EC, Elias K, Mc Cluskey RT, Cooper N. Cryoglobulinemia — A clinical and laboratory study. Am J Med 1966 ; 40 : 837-42.
7. Jori GP, Buonanno G. Chronic hepatitis and cirrhosis of the liver in cryoglobulinemia. Gut 1972 ; 13 : 610-3.
8. Levo Y, Gorevic PD, Kassab HJ, Tobias H, Franklin EC. Liver involvement in the syndrome of mixed cryoglobulinemia. Ann Intern Med 1977 ; 87 : 287-91.
9. Zarski JP, Rougier D, Aubert H, Renversez JC, Cordonnier D, Stoebner P, Rachail M. Association cryoglobuline et maladie hépatique : fréquence, nature et caractères immunochimiques de la cryoglobulinémie. Gastroenterol clin biol 1984 ; 8 : 845-50.
10. Monti G, Navassa G, Fiocca S, Cereda UG, Galli M, Invernizzi F. Cryoglobulinemia and liver involvement. Ric Clin Lab 1986 ; 16 : 367-75.
11. Pascual M, Perrin L, Giostra E, Schifferli JA. HCV in patients with cryoglobulinemia type II. J Infect Dis 1990 ; 162 : 569-70.
12. Ferri C, Greco F, Longombardo G. Association between hepatitis C vius and mixed cryoglubulinemia. Clin Exp Rheumatol 1991 ; 9 : 621-4.
13. Bambara LM, Biasi D, Caramaschi P, Carletto A, Pacor ML. Cryoglobulinemia and hepatitis C virus (HCV) infection. Clin Exp Rheumatol 1991 ; 9 : 96-7.
14. Casato M, Pucillo LP, Lagana B, Taliani G, Goffredo F, Bonomo L. Cryoglobulinaemia and hepatitis C virus. Lancet 1991 ; 337 : 1047-8.
15. Disdier P, Harle JR, Weiller PJ. Cryoglobulinemia and hepatitis C infection. Lancet 1991 ; 338 : 1151-2.
16. Durand JM, Lefèvre P, Harle JR, Boucrat J, Vivitski L, Soubeyrand J. Cutaneous vasculitis and cryoglobulinaemia type II associated with hepatitis C virus infection. Lancet 1991 ; 337 : 499-500.
17. Cacoub P, Musset L, Lunel-Fabiani F, Leger JM, Thi Huong Du L, Piette JC, Godeau P.

Cryoglobulinémies mixtes et hépatite virale C ou que reste-t-il des cryoglobulinémies mixtes « essentielles » ? Rev Méd Interne 1991 ; 12 : 301.
18. Dammacco F, Sansonno D. Antibodies to hepatitis C virus in essential mixed cryoglobulinemia. Clin Exp Immunol 1992 ; 87 : 352-6.
19. Lunel F, Cacoub P, Musset L, Léger JM, Valla D, Perrin M, Frangeul L, Bousquet O, Piette JC, Godeau P, Le Charpentier Y, Opolon P, Huraux JM. Prevalence of hepatitis C virus infection in 115 patients with mixed cryoglobulinemia. Hepatology 1992 ; 16 : 107.
20. Misiani R, Bellavita P, Fenili D, Borelli G, Marchesi D, Massazza M, Vendramin G, Comotti B, Tanzi E, Scudeller G, Zanetti A. Hepatitis C virus infection in patients with essential mixed cryoglobulinemia. Ann Intern Med 1992 ; 117 : 573-7.
21. Agnello V, Chung RT, Kaplan LM. A role for hepatitis C virus infection in type II cryoglobulinemia. N Eng J Med 1992 ; 19 : 1490-5.
22. Marcellin P, Descamps V, Martinot-Peignoux M, Larzul D, Xu , Boyer N, Pham BN, Crickx B, Guillevin L, Belaich S, Erlinger S, Benhamou JP. Cryoglobulinemia with vasculitis associated with hepatitis C virus infection. Gastroenterology 1993 ; 104 : 272-7.
23. Cacoub P, Musset L, Lunel-Fabiani F, Leger JM, Thi Huong Du L, Perrin M, Wechsler B, Piette JC, Godeau P. Hepatitis C virus and essential mixed cryoglobulinemia. British J Rheumatol, 1993 ; 32 : 689-92.
24. Atlas DH, Cardon L, Bunata J. A note on the use of the kagan falling drop proteinometer. Am J Clin Pathol 1943 ; 7 : 21.
25. Griffiths LL, Gilchist L. Cryoglobulinemia in alcoholic cirrhosis. Lancet 1953 ; 264 : 882-4.
26. Monteverde A, Bordin G, Zigrossi P, Monteverde AI, Campanini M, Cadario G. Cryodependent and cryoproducing involvement of organs in type II essential mixed cryoglobulinemia. Ric Clin Lab 1986 ; 16 : 357-66.
27. Garcia-Bragado F, Viliar M, Biosca M, Vilardell M, Jardi R Allende E. Essential mixed cryoglobulinemia and chronic persistent hepatitis. N Eng J Med 1985 ; 312 : 186.
28. Levo Y, Gorevic PD, Kassab HJ, Zucker-Franklin D, Franklin EC. Association between hepatitis B virus and essential mixed cryoglobulinemia. N Engl J Med 1977 ; 296 : 1501-4.
29. Popp JW, Dienstag JL, Wands JR, Block KJ. Essential mixed cryoglobulinemia without evidence for hepatitis B virus infection. Ann Intern Med 1980 ; 92 : 379-83.
30. Galli M, Invernizzi F. Hepatitis B virus and essential mixed cryoglobulinemia. Ann Int Med 1981 ; 95 : 522.
31. Lunel F, Musset L, Cacoub P, Frangeul L, Perrin M, Grippon P, Hoang C, Valla D, Godeau P, Huraux JM, Opolon P. Cryoglobulinemia in liver diseases : role of hepatitis C virus. Gastroenterology 1994 ; 106 : 1291-300.
32. Cacoub P, Lunel-Fabiani F, Musset L, Perrin M, Frangeul L, Galli J, Opolon P, Huraux JM, Piette JC, Godeau P. Mixed cryoglobulinemia and hepatitis C virus. Am J Med 1994 ; 96 : 124-32.
33. Inman RD, Hodge M, Johnston ME, Wricht J, Heathcote J. Arthritis, vasculitis and cryoglobulinemia associated with relapsing hepatitis A virus infection. Ann Intern Med 1986 ; 105 : 700-3.
34. Fiorini G, Bernasconi P, Sinico A, Chianese R, Possi F, D'amico G. Increased frequency of antibodies to ubiquitous viruses in essential mixed cryoglobulinemia. Clin Exp Immunol 1986 ; 64 : 65-70.
35. Nardi G, Zanchetta N, Ragni MC, Saracco A, Castagna A, Galli M. Viral antibodies in serum and cryoprecipitate of patients with essential mixed and secondary cryoglobulinemia. Preliminary results. Ric Clin Lab 1986 ; 16 : 345-8.
36. Dammacco F, Sansonno D, Cornacchiulo V, Mennuni C, Carbone R, Lauletta G, Iacobelli AR, Rizzi R. Hepatitis C virus infection and mixed cryoglobulinemia : a striking association. Int J Clin Lab Res 1993 ; 23 : 45-9.
37. Bonomo L, Casato M, Afeltra A, Caccavo D. Treatment of idiopathic mixed cryoglobulinemia with alpha interferon. Am J Med 1987 ; 83 : 726-30.
38. Casato M, Lagana B, Antonelli G, Dianzani F, Bonomo L. Long-term results of therapy with Interferon-alpha for type II essential mixed cryoglobulinemia. Blood 1991 ; 78 : 3142-7.
39. Durand JM, Kaplanski G, Lefèvre P, Richard MA, Andrac L, Trépo C, Soubeyrand J.

Effects of Interferon-alpha2b on cryoglobulinemia related to hepatitis C virus infection. J Infect Dis 1992 ; 165 : 778-9.
40. Knodell RG, Ishak KG, Black WC, Chen TS, Craig R, Kaplowitz N, Kiernan TW, Wollman J. Formulation and application of a numerical scoring system for assessing histological activity in asymptomatic chronic active hepatitis. Hepatology 1981 ; 1 : 434-5.
41. Musset L, Lunel F, Cacoub P, Lacombe C, Opolon P, Galli J, Aucouturier P. IgG subclass levels in patients with chronic hepatitis C and mixed cryoglobulinemia. International symposium on viral hepatitis and liver disease (Tokyo). 1993 ; P 379 : 190 (Abstract).
42. Mishiro S, Hoshi Y, Takeda K, Yoshikawa A, Gotanda T, Takayashi K, Akahane Y, Yoshikawa H, Okamoto H, Tsuda F, Peterson DA, Muchmore E. Non-A non-B hepatitis specific antibodies directed at host-derived epitope : implication for an autoimmune process. Lancet 1990 ; 336 : 1400-3.

4

HCV genotypes and genotyping methods

L. STUYVER

Department Molecular Biology, Innogenetics NV, Industriepark 7, box 4 B-9052, Gent, Belgium.

Introduction

Like other members of the Togaviridae (Pestiviruses, Flaviviruses), hepatitis C viruses (HCV) are, small enveloped viruses, sensitive to chloroform and containing a singlestranded, positive-sense RNA genome [1, 2]. HCV is the causative agent of most posttransfusion non-A, non-B hepatitis cases. HCV-infected patients very often develop a chronic hepatitis which can result in liver cirrhosis or hepatocellular carcinoma [3].

Although the replication scheme of HCV is not yet completely known, DNA intermediates have never been found. As is the case for the Pesti- and Flaviviruses, the NS5b region encodes a RNA-dependent RNA polymerase (RDRP) [4, 5]. The detected antigenomic (minus) RNA strands, found in liver tissue and in peripheral blood lymphocytes [6, 7], are thought to be the result of the RDRP activity.

In general, the mutation rate of base substitutions for RNA viruses is roughly 10^3 times as high as for DNA viruses and 10^6 times as high as the frequency observed in mammals [8]. These base substitutions are random mutations incorporated by the viral RDRP, and are neutral, which means that they are neither advantageous nor disadvantageous [9]. However, the natural selection against deleterious or nonfunctional mutants, accounting for the conservation of biologically significant sequences, cannot be ruled out. The HCV genome would therefore drift continuously and randomly, but non-randomly at the species level.

This capacity of variation incorporation enables HCV to escape from the host's immune system. This is demonstrated by the genetic drift observed in the envelope E1 and E2 region during the course of a chronic infection [10]. The overall mutation rate of the E2 region was estimated to be 2.7×10^3 base substitutions per site per year. However, the mutation rate was reduced to 0 and 0.41×10^3 base substitutions per site per year for the 5' untranslated region (UR) and the NS4b region, respectively. This reduction in mutation rate could possibly be explained by assuming that most of the (non-synonymous) mutations are lethal to the virus, whereas they are tolerated in the hypervariable regions of the viral envelope proteins. The overall mutation rate was estimated as 1.92×10^3 (H-strain) and 1.44×10^3 (HC-J4 strain) base substitutions per site per year [10, 11]. Thus, *in vivo*, HCV exists as a population of slightly different viruses, representing a collective identity which is known as the quasispecies [12].

HCV genotypes

Starting from the putative HCV-like ancestor, this rapid evolution finally resulted in the existence of so called « types », « subtypes », and « isolates or strains belonging to the same subtype ». The high degree of sequence heterogeneity has led to considerable confusion with respect to nomenclature. A convenient classification system has now been widely accepted by most scientists in the HCV variability field [13].

At present, 6 major groups or « types » have been described with an overall homology of less than 69 % between members of the different types. Each type can contain from one to several clearly separated subgroups or « subtypes ». Isolates belonging to different subtypes of the same type are about 79 % homologous. Finally, individual isolates belonging to the same subtype show a sequence similarity of more than 88 %. The six major genotypes are composed of at least 16 subtypes, namely : 1a, 1b, 1c, 2a, 2b, 2c, 3a, 3b, 4a, 4b, 4c, 4d, 4e, 4f, 5a, and 6a. Fourteen complete genomes confirmed the existence of types, subtypes and isolates (EMBL accession numbers for type 1a : M62321, M67463, D10749 ; for type 1b : D90208, M58335, D01217 and D10750, D01171 and D01172 and S38204, L02836, M84754, X61596, M96362, S62220 ; for type 2a : D00944 ; for type 2b : D10899 and D01221).

Because of the difficulties in determining complete HCV genomes, most researchers have only analyzed shorter fragments, especially : the 5' UR [14] ; the regions starting at the initiating methionine of the core protein until the highly conserved 3-methionine stretch in the envelope protein E1 (amino acid positions 1-322) [14-16] ; complete E1 [17] ; or the 401 bp NS5b sequence obtained with the primers first described by Enomoto [16, 18, 19]. The assignment of a certain genotype to such a partial HCV sequence can only be reliable if it is compared with the corresponding regions of the prototype isolates (preferably complete genomes), both at the sequence homology and phylogenetic analysis level [13]. If the genotype assignment is based on only one region, it is advisable to confirm this with another region. All entries of partial HCV genomes (nearly 600) in the EMBL database, release 36, fit into this system of nomenclature.

Genotype distribution

The distribution of the different genotypes varies from country to country. HCV type 1, 2, and 3 have been found in almost all countries tested, including Europe [20, 21], North America [17, 22], South America [20] and eastern Asia [23, 24]. Type 4 was mainly found in Africa and in the Middle East [14, 19, 20], but is also present at lower percentages in Europe [20, 21]. Type 5, which was originally described for South Africa [17, 25], was also found in Europe and central Africa [20]. Type 6 has only been found in serum samples originating from Hong Kong [17, 19, 25].

Based on the analysis of 123 Belgian samples, up to 58 % of the infections were caused by genotype 1b, while only 8 % of 1a was found. Type 2a was represented by 8 % of infections, while type 2b occured in less than 1 %. The prevalences of type 3a, 4, and 5 were 17 %, 5 %, and 3 %, respectively [20]. Genotype 1b was detected in up to 81 % of interferon-treated chronic patients. A comparable distribution was found in the Netherlands [21].

In Brazil, the following prevalences were found in 114 samples tested : type 1a 42 %, type 1b 34 %, type 2a 2 %, type 2b 1 %, type 3a 19 %, and 2 % co-infections of type 1 and 3. Types 4 or 5 were never detected.

In China, 77 % type 1b and 31 % type 2a was found ; no type 1a, type 2b, or types 3, 4 or 5 infections were described. However, high region-dependent fluctuations in the above percentages were reported [26].

In Japan, 5 % type 1a, 80 % type 1b, 10 % 2a, and 5 % 2b was found in blood donors. According to the population under study (blood donors, patients, hemophiliacs), these distributions varied strongly. For example, an increased percentage of types 1a and 3 and a decreased percentage of types 1b and 2a were found in hemophiliacs when compared with the percentages from blood donors [26].

In Gabon (central Africa) 48 % of the sera tested contained a type 4 genotype, 10 % type 5, 3 % type 1a, 3 % 1b, and 5 % type 2a. Up to 31 % could not be genotyped [20].

HCV genotyping methods

It is very likely that all the different genotypes which have been identified contain different antigenic properties, which in turn can have important consequences for vaccine development [27]. It was also proven that immunoreactive regions like NS4 and E1 express type-specific epitopes [16, 28, 29], thus influencing the effectiveness of antibody screenings and confirmation assays. Also, the severity of the disease [30], the amount of viral particals present in the patient serum [31], and the susceptibility and response to interferon treatment [32-34] can be influenced largely by the type and/or subtype of infection. It is therefore important to recognize the different types and subtypes of HCV.

Traditionally, viruses have been grouped into serotypes. Attempts have already been undertaken to classify the major genotypes into serological types [16, 28, 35]. These results are mostly ambiguous. Further research is needed before serotyping becomes widely available and, although subtyping is clinically significant, serological subtyping may prove impossible [29].

Several genotyping methods, based on restriction fragment length polymorphism analysis (RFLP) [36, 37], type-specific PCR [24, 38, 39] or reverse hybridization have been described [41]. RFPL analysis was established for the NS5b region and for the 5' UR region. In the NS5b region, a 401-bp PCR fragment can be generated by means of a very highly conserved set of primers [18] from all six genotypes. The method to classify the HCV genomes in this region was demonstrated for the type 1 and 2 genotypes using the AccI, Sau96I and AluI restriction enzymes [36]. This kind of RFLP analysis was further extended for types 3, 4, 5, and 6 in the 5' UR [14, 36, 37] with the restriction enzymes Sau3a, HaeIII, RsaI, ScrfI and HinfI. Subtyping for types 1 and 2 was possible in the NS5 region, but becomes nearly impossible in the 5' UR. A double restriction analysis is often required to discriminate between types.

Another method used type-specific PCR primers for HCV typing. This procedure was elaborated for the NS5b region [38] and for the core region [24, 39]. For the NS5 region, a first round PCR was generated with the Enomoto primers [18]. This 401-bp PCR fragment was than subjected to a nested PCR with mixed subtype-specific primers. A PCR fragment of subtype-specific size was generated. After gel electrophoresis, the subtype could be determined according to the observed size [38]. This procedure allows the recognition of genotypes 1a, 1b, 2a, and 2b. Based on the same principle, a genotyping assay was established in the core region [24, 39], allowing detection of genotypes 1a, 1b, 2a, 2b, and 3a. A first-round PCR fragment of 276-bp was generated with a mixture of highly conserved primers (two sense primers and one antisense primer). Second-round PCR with mixtures of subtype-specific primers again generated subtype-specific amplification products. The best results are obtained when each HCV subtype is separately amplified [40]. A high amount of 1a and 1b co-infections is very often found by using the nested subtype 1a antisense primer 132 (sometimes up to 20 %). This primer can be theoretically predicted to hybridize to many subtype 1b sequences. Normally, two mismatches lead to the difference between both subtypes at the primer 132 position. However, isolates HPCUNKCDS and HCV-N (EMBL accession numbers M96362, S62220), two complete subtype 1b genomes, only differ by one variation. Due to aspecific priming of primer 132, it is possible that both isolates are recognized as a co-infection. The introduction of the nested subtype 1a antisense primer 296 (with up to 5 mismatches against the subtype 1b) [24, 26] should reduce the number of detected co-infections to more realistic proportions (1-3 %).

Because of the increasing number of types and subtypes, and the higher variability in the core and NS5 region compared with the variability in the 5' UR, updating of the above-mentioned genotyping assays is no longer tenable. An alternative genotyping assay which allows quick adaptations to include the detection of newly discovered genotypes is offered by the Line Probe Assay (LiPA) [41].

The LiPA is a reverse hybridization assay based on highly conserved variations in the 5' UR. The current LiPA allows typing and subtyping of the most common genotypes 1a, 1b, 2a, 2b, 3a, 4, and 5. Essentially, a cPCR fragment is synthesized from the 5' UR of any HCV genome using sets of primers targeting highly conserved regions. The oligonucleotides used for (sub)typing are directed against internal variable parts, more precisely between positions − 170 and − 155 and between − 132 and − 117. After hybridization of the biotinylated cPCR fragments to the immobilized (sub)typing probes, streptavidin labelled with alkaline phosphatase is added and becomes bound to any previously formed biotinylated hybrid. Incubation with NBT and BCIP chromogen results in a purple brown precipitate. The INNOLiPA has been proven to be a reliable system [16, 20, 21, 29]. It is not known whether the signature sequence of the 5' UR, used to design the typing probes, will invariably appear in all HCV strains. Up to now, no exceptions to these motifs have been found. Subtyping in the 5' UR is mostly based on only one variation, for example at position − 99 for type 1a/1b, and positions − 161 and − 124 for type 2a/2b. Analysis of the genotype 1a and 1b strains entered in the EMBL database, for which also part of the coding region is known, predicted that 8 % of these would be mistyped. It is therefore necessary to carefully evaluate this variation in larger groups of type 1 HCV strains. Also, the sensitivity for detecting co-infections needs to be further investigated.

Applications of the LiPA in the search for new genotypes

The LiPA is provided with a pair of universal HCV probes. Positive reactions on those control probes in combination with the absence or aberrancy of staining on typing probes is mostly indicative for new genotypes. In the case of the serum samples from Gabon, up to 31 % were only reactive with the control probes [20]. Before a specific genotype could be assigned to these sera, sequence information was gathered from the core/E1 region, NS5b region and the 5' UR, regions which are usually used in comparative studies.

The relationship between newly obtained sequences with prototype isolates could either be expressed as a percentage of homology or as a phylogenetic distance. Phylogenetic analysis takes into account the possibility of multiple substitutions at each position. Homology calculations therefore greatly underestimate the true extent of divergence. The DNADIST program from the PHYLIP package [42] directly provides these molecular evolutionary distances. According to this DNADIST matrix, and based on 800 pairwise comparisons, a gap was found between the ranges of evolutionary distances from isolates and subtypes, and between those from subtypes and types. This gap was present after analysis of both the core/E1 region and in the NS5b region. For the core/E1 region, minimum and maximum values were 0.0402 – 0.111 (average 0.0772 ; SD ± 0.0197) for isolates belonging to the same subtype, 0.1864 – 0.3535 (0.2833 ; SD ± 0.0350) for isolates belonging to different subtypes and 0.3824 – 0.6230 (0.4894 ; SD ± 0.0554) for isolates belonging to different types. In the NS5 region, these values ranged from 0.0148 to 0.1064 (0.0623 ; SD ± 0.0181) for isolates belonging to the same subtype, from 0.1384 to 0.2675 (0.2312 ; SD ± 0.0182) for isolates belonging to different subtypes, and from 0.3581 to 0.6549 (0.4942 ; SD ± 0.0485) for isolates belonging to different types.

After calculating the phylogenetic distances from the Gabonese HCV strains against the prototype sequences and type 4 E1 sequences [17], it became clear that the newly obtained sequences belonged to type 4. Based on the previously calculated phylogenetic border distances, type 4 HCV strains could be split up into at least 6 subtypes (4a to 4f) [43]. Most of the new type 4 subtypes again contained signature sequences in the 5' UR. Adaptations of the LiPA should allow the recognition of those different type 4 subtypes, enabling the study of their prevalence in other countries.

Conclusion

Hepatitis C virus is a rapid evolving, single-stranded RNA virus, which exists *in vivo* as a quasispecies. At this moment six major genotypes and at least 16 subtypes have been described. HCV genotypes 1, 2, and 3 were found in almost all countries. Type 4 and 5 were most prevalent in Africa, but were also found in Europe in lower percentages. Type 6 seems to be unique for Hong Kong. Assignment of a certain genotype to newly obtained sequences can be reliable done after homology and phylogenetic distance calculation against core/E1 and NS5b prototype sequences.

The demonstration that different HCV genotype infections result in different serological reactivities and response to interferon treatment stresses the importance of HCV genotyping. At least three different genotyping approaches, either based on RFLP analysis, subtype-specific amplifications, or reverse hybridization, have been described. In particular, the use of the LiPA allows an easy detection of new types and/or subtypes. This was demonstrated with serum samples originating from Gabon.

Acknowledgements : we had to acknowledge Dr. Geert Maertens for critically reviewing and Mr. Fred Shapiro for improving and editing the text.

References

1. Bradley DW, McCaustland KA, Cook EH, Schable CA, Ebert JW, Maynard JE. Post-transfusion non-A, non-B hepatitis in chimpanzees. Physicochemical evidence that the tubule-forming agent is a small, enveloped virus. Gastroenterology 1985 ; 88 : 773-9.
2. Miller RH, Purcell RH. Hepatitis C virus shares amino acid sequence similarity with pestiviruses and flaviviruses as well as members of two plant virus supergroups. Proc Natl Acad Sci USA. 1990 ; 87 : 2057-61.
3. Takahashi M, Yamada G, Miyamoto R, Doi T, Endo H, Tsuji T. Natural course of chronic hepatitis. Am J Gastroenterology 1993 ; 88 : 240-3.
4. Koonin EV. The phylogeny of RNA-dependant RNA polymerases of positive-strand RNA viruses. J Gen Virol 1991 ; 72 : 2197-206.
5. Chung RT, Kaplan LM. Isolation and characterization of an HCV-specific RNA dependent RNA polymerase activity in extracts of infected liver tissue. In : Hepatitis C virus and related viruses. 1st annual meeting Venice 1992 A15 (abstract).
6. Takahare T, Hayasi N, Mita E, *et al.* Detection of minus strand of hepatitis C virus RNA by reverse transcription and polymerase chain reaction : implication for hepatitis C virus replication in infected tissue. Hepatology 1992 ; 15 : 387-90.
7. Fong TL, Shindo M, Feinstone SM, Hoofnagle JH, DiBisceglie AM. Detection of replicative intermediates of Hepatitis C viral RNA in liver and serum of patients with chronic hepatitis C. J Clin Invest 1991 ; 88 : 1058-60.
8. Gojobori T, Moriyama EN, Kimura M. Molecular clock of viral evolution, and the neutral theory. Proc Natl Acad Sci USA 1990 ; 87 : 10015-8.
9. Kimura M. The neutral theory of molecular evolution. Cambridge University Press, Cambridge, England, 1983.
10. Okamoto H, Kojima M, Okada SI, *et al.* Genetic drift of hepatitis C virus during an 8.2 year infection in a chimpanzee : variability and stability. Virology 1992 ; 190 : 894-9.
11. Ogata N, Alter HJ, Miller RH, Purcell RH. Nucleotide sequence and mutation rate of the H strain of hepatitis C virus. Proc Natl Acad Sci USA 1991 ; 88 : 3392-6.
12. Martell M, Esteban JI, Quer J, *et al.* Hepatitis C virus (HCV) circulates as a population of different but closely related genomes : quasispecies nature of HCV genome distribution. J Virol 1992 ; 3225-9.
13. Simmonds P, Alberti A, Bonino F, *et al.* Nomenclature for genotypes of Hepatitis C Virus. Hepatology 1994, in press.

14. Simmonds P, McOmish F, Yap PL, Chan S-W, Lin CK, Dusheiko G, Saeed AA, Holmes EC. Sequence variability in the 5'non-coding region of hepatitis C virus : identification of a new virus type and restrictions on sequence diversity. J Gen Virol 1993 ; 74 : 661-8.
15. Chayama K, Tsubota A, Arase Y. Unpublished. JDDB accession number D11443.
16. Stuyver L, Van Arnhem W, Wyseur A, DeLeys R, Maertens G. Analysis of the putative E1 envelope and NS4a epitope regions of HCV type 3. Biochem Biophys Res Commun 1993 ; 192 : 635-41.
17. Bukh J, Purcell RH, Miller RH. At least 12 genotypes of hepatitis C virus predicted by sequence analysis of the putative E1 gene of isolates collected worldwide. Proc Natl Acad Sci USA 1993 ; 90 : 8234-38.
18. Enomoto N, Takada A, Nakao T, Date T. There are two major types of hepatitis C virus in Japan. Biochem Biophys Res Commun 190 ; 170 : 1021-5.
19. Simmonds P, Holmes EC, Cha T-A, et al. Classification of hepatitis C virus into six major genotypes and a series of subtypes by phylogenetic analysis of the NS5 region. J Gen Virol 74 : 2391-9.
20. Stuyver L, Wyseur A, Van Arnhem W, et al. The use of a Line Probe Assay as a tool to detect new types or subtypes of the hepatitis C virus. In : Viral Hepatitis and Liver Disease, Proceedings of the 1993 International Symposium on Viral Hepatitis and Liver Disease (Eds. Suzuki et al.), in press.
21. Van Doorn LJ, Kleter GEM, Stuyver L, et al. Analysis of hepatitis C virus genotypes by a line probe assay (LiPA) and correlation with antibody profiles. J Hepatol, in press.
22. Lee C-H, Cheng C, Wang J, Lumeng L. Identification of hepatitis C viruses with a non-conserved sequence of the 5' untranslated region. J Clin Microbiol 1992 ; 1602-4.
23. Mori S, Kato N, Yagyu A, et al. A new type of hepatitis C virus in patients in Thailand. Biochem Biophys Res Commun 1992 ; 183 : 334-42.
24. Okamoto H, Tokita H, Sakamoto M, Horikita M, Kojima M, Iizuka H, Mishiro S. Characterization of the genomic sequence of type V (or 3a) hepatitis C virus isolates and PCR primers for specific detection. J Gen Virol 1993 ; 74 : 2385-90.
25. Cha T-A, Beal E, Irvine B, Kolberg J, Chien D, Kuo G, Urdea MS. At least five related but distinct hepatitis C viral genotypes exist. Proc Natl Acad Sci USA 1992 ; 89 : 7144-8.
26. Kinoshita T, Miyake K, Okamoto h, Mishiro S. Imported hepatitis C virus genotypes in Japanese hemophiliacs. J Inf Dis 1993 ; 168 : 249-50.
27. Farci P, Alter HJ, Govindarajan S, et al. Lack of protective immunity against reinfection with hepatitis C virus. Science 1992 ; 258 : 135-40.
28. Simmonds P, Rose KA, Graham S, et al. Mapping of serotype-specific, immunodominant epitopes in the NS4 region of hepatitis C virus (HCV) : Use of type-specific peptides to serologically differentiate infections with HCV types 1, 2, and 3. J Clin Microbiol 1993 ; 31 : 1493-503.
29. Maertens G, Ducatteeuw A, Stuyver L, et al. Low prevalence of anti-E1 antibodies reactive to recombinant type 1b E1 envelope protein in type 2, 3, and 4 HCV sera, but high prevalence in subtype 1a and 1b. In : Viral Hepatitis and Liver Disease, Proceedings of the 1993 International Symposium on Viral Hepatitis and Liver Disease (Eds. Suzuki et al.), in press.
30. Silini E, Bono F, Cividini A, Cerino A, Civardi E, Mondelli MU. High prevalence of Hepatitis C virus genotype III infection in patients with normal liver enzymes and mild histological lesions. Hepatology 1993 ; 18 : No 4, Pt.2, AASLD abstract 83A, 107.
31. Yotsuyanagi H, Yasuda K, Koike K, Moriya K, Hino K, Iino S, Kurokawa K. Genotypes and quantity of genome in Chronic hepatitis C infection. In : International Symposium on Viral Hepatitis and Liver Disease, Tokyo 1993 ; Abstract 324.
32. Pozatto G, Moretti M, Franzin F, et al. Severity of liver disease with different hepatitis C viral clones. Lancet 1991 ; 338 : 509.
33. Kanai K, Kako M, Okamoto H. HCV genotypes in chronic hepatitis C and response to interferon. Lancet 1992 ; 339 : 1543.

34. Yoshioka K, Kakumu S, Wakita T, et al. Detection of hepatitis C virus by polymerase chain reaction and response to interferon-à therapy : relationship to genotypes of hepatitis C virus. Hepatology 1992 ; 16 : 293-9.
35. Machida A, Ohnuma H, Tsuda F, Munekata E, Tanaka T, Akahane Y, Okamoto H, Mishiro S. Two distinct subtypes of hepatitis C virus defined by antibodies directed to the putative core protein. Hepatology 1992 ; 16 : 886-91.
36. Nakao T, Enomoto N, Takada N, Takada A, Date T. Typing of hepatitis C virus genomes by restriction length polymorphism. J Gen Virol 1991 ; 72 : 2105-12.
37. Dusheiko G, Schmilovitz-Weiss H, Brown D, et al. Hepatitis C virus : An investigation of type specific differences in geographic origin and disease. Hepatology 1994 ; 19 : 13-8.
38. Kurosaki M, Enomoto N, Marumo F, Sato C. Rapid sequence variation of the hypervariable region of hepatitis C virus during the course of chronic infection. Hepatology 1993 ; 18 : 1293-9.
39. Okamoto H, Sugiuama Y, Okada SI, et al. Typing hepatitis C virus by polymerase chain reaction with type-specific primers : application to clinical surveys and tracing infectious sources. J Gen Virol 1992 ; 73 : 673-9.
40. Kobayashi Y, Watanabe S, Konishi M, et al. Quantitiation and typing of serum hepatitis C virus RNA in patients with chronic hepatitis C treated with interferon-β. Hepatology 1993 ; 18 : 1319-25.
41. Stuyver L, Rossau R, Wyseur A, Duhamel M, Vanderborght B, Van Heuverswyn H, Maertens G. Typing of hepatitis C virus isolates and characterization of new subtypes using a line probe assay. J Gen Virol 1993 ; 74 : 1093-102.
42. Felsenstein J. PHYLIP (Phylogeny Inference Package) version 3.5c. 1993. Distributed by the author. Department of Genetics, University of Washington, Seattle, USA.
43. Stuyver L, Delaporte E, Van Arnhem W, Wyseur A, Hernandez F, Maertens G. Classification of hepatitis C viruses based on phylogenetic analysis of the core/E1, NS3/NS4 and NS5b regions and discovery of new subtypes in genotype 2 and 4. Manuscript in preparation.

5

Multicentre quality control of hepatitis C virus RNA polymerase chain reaction

J.-J. LEFRÈRE[1]
on behalf of the Groupe Français d'Études Moléculaires des Hépatites (GEMHEP)[2]

[1] *Institut National de Transfusion Sanguine, Hôpital Saint-Antoine, Paris, France.*

The Hepatitis C virus (HCV) was discovered in 1989 and has been recognized as the main agent of post-transfusional non A, non B hepatitis [1]. Serological assays applicable in the routine diagnosis of the infection [2] were made possible by the sequencing of the HCV genome. However, the evidencing of viral RNA through polymerase chain reaction (PCR) [3] remains necessary to affirm the infection in a certain number of cases [4]. Indeed, PCR is a highly sensitive technique for detection of viral RNAs such as HCV in serum [5]. Viremia may be detected through PCR within only a few days of exposure to the virus and several weeks before elevation of serum alanine aminotransferase activity and anti-HCV antibody levels [6]. Valuable information concerning the infectious status when anti-HCV antibodies are present but liver function is normal can be provided through PCR [7]. Furthermore, PCR is helpful to monitor therapeutic efficacy [8] and to diagnose HCV infection in chronic non A, non B hepa-

[2] *Laboratoire de virologie transfusionnelle, Institut National de Transfusion Sanguine, Paris (Françoise Bouchardeau) ; Centre Régional de Transfusion Sanguine, Lille (Christine Defer) ; Laboratoire de virologie, Services des maladies du foie et de l'appareil digestif, Hôpital de Bicêtre, Le Kremlin-Bicêtre (Elisabeth Dussaix, Pierre Laurent-Puig) ; Laboratoire d'immunologie, Hôpital St-Antoine (Jean-Claude Homberg) ; Hôpital Louis-Mourier, Colombes (Jérôme Lamoril, Marie-France Fruchard) ; Institut National de Transfusion Sanguine, Hôpital St-Antoine, Paris (Jean-Jacques Lefrère, Martine Mariotti) ; Laboratoire Cerba, Cergy-Pontoise (Patricia Lewin) ; Centre de Transfusion, Hôpital St-Louis, Paris (Pascale Loiseau, Nadine Ravera) ; Service de bactériologie-virologie, Hôpital de la Pitié-Salpétrière, Paris (Françoise Lunel, Lionel Frangeul) ; Unité d'hépatologie, Hôpital Beaujon, Clichy (Patrick Marcellin, Michèle Martinot-Peignoux) ; Laboratoire de bactério-virologie, Hôpital Henri-Mondor, Créteil (Jean-Michel Pawlotsky) ; Centre de Transfusion, Hôpital Foch, Suresnes (Dominique Vignon) ; Laboratoire de Virologie, Centre Hospitalo-Universitaire, Grenoble (Jean-Pierre Zarski, Annette Ounanian).*

titis patients who may be serologically negative or not conclusive, in particular for immunodepressed individuals. PCR is also useful to early detect HCV infection in patients having received organ grafts. Finally, PCR is of particular interest in the study of materno-foetal transmission of HCV [9, 10].

The importance of the parameters influencing the sensitivity and specifity of PCR has been underlined, in particular the conditions of use of the Taq polymerase [11], the localisation of the primers [12, 13] or the extraction methods of viral RNA [14]. Because of its high sensitivity, PCR can generate false-positive results [15] usually due to laboratory contamination or DNA carryover. Technical problems in PCR procedure can also be responsible for false-negative results. Strict guidelines on sample preparation, PCR conditions and evidence of amplified products are therefore required, and PCR procedures should generally be standardized among laboratories. The realisation of multicentre quality controls is thus indispensable.

A recently published international quality control study (« Eurohep ») reported important discrepancies in results obtained by the 31 participating laboratories with a coded panel including 4 HCV positive plasma samples and 6 HCV negative plasma samples, and two dilution series of HCV positive plasma [16] ; 10 (32 %) laboratories had faultless results with undiluted plasma samples ; 15 (48 %) reported correct results with both dilution series. Only 5 laboratories (16 %) performed faultlessly with the entire panel, but reported a hundred-fold difference in sensitivity for the dilution series. In this study, the obtention of correct results was not associated with a particular RNA-extraction method, with nested PCR or with detection by hybridisation. The authors concluded that PCR studies should include negative controls to monitor contamination and weak positive samples to guarantee sensitivity of the procedure.

Nine French laboratories, using reverse nested PCR for detection of HCV RNA, initiated a multicentre quality control study [17] not only to assess the specificity and sensitivity of their PCR procedures but also to determine optimal PCR conditions for the detection of HCV RNA with maximum diagnosis proficiency and to allow each participating laboratory to improve its own procedure. The quality control study was performed in three successive rounds, based on three different panels (detailed in Table I), each consisting of samples obtained from the following groups of individuals : Group A (positive

Table I. Constitution of the three panels used in the French multicentre quality control. Group A (positive controls) comprised samples from anti-HCV positive individuals (on Elisa-2 and Riba-2) ; group B (negative controls) comprised samples from anti-HCV negative individuals at low risk of HCV infection.

	group A	group B
Panel 1	8	5
Panel 2	9	5
Panel 3	5*	3

* Three of the positive controls were mixed into the negative controls at the following dilutions : 1/10, 1/100, 1/1,000, 1/10,000.

controls) comprised anti-HCV positive individuals. Diagnosis of HCV infection was based on a positive second generation (Elisa-2), with validation by a second generation Riba (Riba-2) simultaneously evidencing at least two different antibodies. No individual was positive for hepatitis B antigen through specific radio-immunoassay and for HIV through specific Elisa. All had a serum alanine aminotransferase activity higher than twice the norm, a chronic active hepatitis on liver biopsy and no other cause of liver disease. None had as yet received interferon therapy. Group B (negative controls) comprised anti-HCV negative (on Elisa-2 and Riba-2) individuals at low risk of HCV infection. Patients from groups A and B were different at each panel. Certain samples were duplicated without informing the laboratories how many were in group A and group B. To blindly perform PCR, panels 1, 2 and 3 were prepared, coded and supplied by an investigator external to the participating laboratories. Decoding of laboratory results was performed by the same investigator external to the participating laboratories. Laboratories were identified with a letter (established by a random draw) unconnected to our author list.

First round used panel 1 (Table I). Blood was collected on lithium heparinate, 2 500 U/ml. After centrifugation at 4 °C at 1 500 rpm during 10 min, the plasmas obtained were aliquoted and stored at - 70 °C. Each laboratory followed its own protocol for RNA extraction, cDNA synthesis and nested PCR, and used its own primer pairs. Results obtained on panel 1 are given in Table II : 100 % sensitivity (defined as the percentage of positive PCR results in samples collected from group A individuals) was observed in two of the nine laboratories (22 %), and 100 % specificity (defined as the percentage of negative PCR results in samples collected from group B individuals) in 7 laboratories (77 %). One laboratory had both 100 % sensitivity

Table II. PCR results of participating laboratoires for panel 1 (tested with personal procedure) and panel 2 (tested with personal procedure (PP) and common procedure (CP)). Primer pairs used in panel 1 are given in Table I. Common primer pairs used in panel 2 were SR1/SF1, SR2/SF2. Personal primer pairs used in panel 2 were the same as those used in panel 1 for laboratories E, F, I, J, L, O, Q ; laboratoires B and K, performing a one-stage PCR to assay panel 2, used NCR 1/2 and KB3/KB4, respectively.

Laboratories	B	E	F	I	J	K	L	O	Q
Panel 1									
Number of positive results	9	7	0	6	2	8	8	8	7
Group A* (n = 8)	8	7	0	6	2	7	7	8	7
Group B* (n = 5)	1	0	0	0	0	1	0	0	0
Concordance with serology (%)**	93	93	38	84	54	84	93	100	92
Sensitivity (%)	100	88	0	75	25	88	88	100	88
Specificity (%)	80	100	100	100	100	80	100	100	100

Panel 2	B CP	B PP	E CP	E PP	F CP	F PP	I CP	I PP	J CP	J PP	K CP	K PP	L CP	L PP	O CP	O PP	Q CP	Q PP
Number of positive results	9	9	9	9	4	5	9	8	9	9	NT	NT	9	9	8	9	9	9
Group A (n = 9)	9	9	9	8	4	5	9	8	9	9	NT	NT	9	9	8	9	9	9
Group B (n = 5)	0	0	0	0	0	0	0	0	0	0	NT	NT	0	0	0	0	0	0
Concordance with serology (%)**	100	100	100	93	64	71	100	93	100	100	NT	NT	100	100	93	100	100	100
Sensitivity (%)	100	100	100	89	44	55	100	89	100	100	NT	NT	100	100	89	100	100	100
Specificity (%)	100	100	100	100	100	100	100	100	100	100	NT	NT	100	100	100	100	100	100

* See text for definition of groups A and B.
** Concordance [(HCV-seropositive/PCR+) + (HCV-seronegative/PCR-)/Total results] × 100.
NT = non tested.

and 100 % specificity. The false-negative and false-positive PCR results were not observed for the same samples, indicating that such results were linked rather to cross-contaminations than to DNA carryover.

The nine participating laboratories of our group had identical differences of sensitivity (0 to 100 %) and specificity (80 to 100 %) when studying panel 1. The causes of such differences could be : extraction conditions, choice of primer pairs, amplification conditions not optimized (such as magnesium concentration, temperature and time of PCR steps), as evidenced by the differences between laboratories shown by the detailed questionnaire used to establish the common procedure. However, a comparison of the PCR procedures used in the participating laboratories to assay panel 1 allowed to exclude some factors that might have been responsible for false-positive and false-negative signals in the study of this panel. The amount of cDNA tested, ranged from

5 to 20 µl according to the different laboratories, did not appear to affect PCR sensitivity within these limits. The different quantities of enzymes (reverse transcriptase and Taq polymerase) and the number of cycles appeared to be equally efficient.

After the first round, two possibilities existed to attain better results for the whole of the group : first, to improve the deficient steps in the specific PCR procedure of each participating laboratory ; second, to establish a validated and standardized PCR procedure which could be used to initiate laboratories to this assay. These two aims were realised during the second round. After decoding of the panel 1 results, the PCR procedures of the participating laboratories were compared by means of a detailed questionaire, in order to assay the panel 2 samples with a common procedure established from that of the laboratories which provided the best results on panel 1. Panel 2 is detailed in Table I. For this second panel, the serum was prefered to plasma because an inhibiting effect of lithium heparinate has been described [18]. After a 1500 rpm centrifugation at 4 °C for 10 min, the sera were aliquoted and stored at - 70 °C. The panel 2 samples were duplicated to allow each laboratory to perform both personal and common PCR procedures. The common procedure, which included imposed primer pairs, is detailed elsewhere [17]. Due to the risk of laboratory contaminations, the different steps of the PCR procedure were performed in separate rooms, and all transfers were made with positive displacement disposable pipettes. The different laboratories included internal known positive and negative controls in each PCR run. Results obtained on panel 2 are given in Table II. With personal PCR procedure, 100 % sensitivity was observed in 5 of the 9 laboratories (55 %) and 100 % specificity in all laboratories (100 %). Five laboratories (55 %) thus had both 100 % sensitivity and 100 % specificity. For the others, discrepancies in PCR results were due to lack of sensitivity. Laboratories E, F, I, J, L used the same personal PCR procedure in both panels. Laboratories K, O and Q modified their procedure to use guanidinium isothiocyanate [14] instead of SDS-proteinase K to extract RNA. Laboratories B and K used a one-stage PCR with an increased number of cycles (forty). With common PCR procedure (applied in 8 of the 9 participating laboratories), 100 % sensitivity was observed in 7 of the 8 laboratories, and 100 % specificity in all laboratories. Seven laboratories had both 100 % sensitivity and 100 % specificity.

Results of panel 2 indicated a strong reduction of the variability of both sensitivity and specificity when laboratories used their own technique which they could have improved when they felt it necessary (5/9 laboratories had 100 % sensitivity and specificity with their own procedure, which could be as of then considered as validated). Furthermore, the results of panel 2 indicated that the majority of the participating laboratories have reached 100 % specificity and 100 % sensitivity with the consensus procedure, allowing certain participating laboratories to adopt this latter procedure in replacement of their own procedure (furthermore, this common procedure became the one our group advised to laboratories preparing themselves to initiate HCV-RNA PCR). No false-positive results were observed in any laboratories during this second round with both procedures, as opposed to the previous round, suggesting that the problems of cross-contaminations had been resolved in participating laboratories.

There remained to further appreciate the differences in sensitivity of PCR assay among the participating laboratories by using diluted samples. It was the aim of the third round. Panel 3 (Table I) was constituted to study the sensitivity of PCR procedure in evidencing weak quantities of HCV RNA in serum. Each participating laboratory could apply either the common PCR procedure used to assay panel 2, either its own PCR procedure as improved by the previous rounds ; 8 from the 9 laboratories assayed this panel. All laboratories had 100 % sensitivity and 100 % specificity with undiluted positive and negative controls, except laboratory I which gave a false-positive result. When considering the three diluted samples, the negative results were observed only for the greater dilutions in all laboratories, except for one sample in one laboratory (see Table III). For samples 1 and 2, 8/8 laboratories had positive PCR signals until the 1/100 dilution ; 6/8 and 7/8 laboratories found samples 1 and 2 positive at 1/1,000 dilution, respectively ; 2/8 and 1/8 laboratories found samples 1 and 2 positive at 1/10,000 dilution, respectively ; for sample 3, the results were more discrepant between the laboratories than for samples 1 and 2, one laboratory reporting negative results at each studied dilution. The results of this third round confirmed the good specificity and sensitivity of the majority of laboratories and validated the methodology of the study. PCR signals of one of the three diluted samples of this panel (sample 3, see Table III) were more discrepant between laboratories than signals from the two others. It could be hypothesized that such difference was linked to the random distribution of a sample with a low HCV-RNA concentration ; indeed, serum HCV RNA concentration of the three samples was quantitated by branched DNA signal amplification (Chiron Diagnostic, Lyon, France) [19] in one laboratory of our group : RNA concentration was 107, 66 and 14.9 × 10^5 equivalents/mL for samples 1, 2 and 3, respectively.

Table III. PCR results of panel 3. Three samples (1, 2, 3) from positive controls were studied through PCR assay after different dilutions (1/10, 1/100, 1/1,000, 1/10,000).

Laboratories	B	F	I	J	K	L	O	Q
Sample 1								
1/10	+	+	+	+	+	+	+	+
1/100	+	+	+	+	+	+	+	+
1/1,000	+	+	+	−	+	−	+	+
1/10,000	+	−	−	−	+	−	−	−
Sample 2 :								
1/10	+	+	+	+	+	+	+	+
1/100	+	+	+	+	+	+	+	+
1/1,000	+	+	+	+	+	+	−	+
1/10,000	−	−	−	−	+	−	−	−
Sample 3 :								
1/10	+	+	+	−	+	+	+	+
1/100	−	+	+	−	+	+	+	+
1/1,000	+	−	+	−	+	+	−	−
1/10,000	+	−	−	−	−	−	−	−

The aim of this quality control of HCV-RNA PCR was to evaluate sensitivity and specificity of each participating laboratory, in order to improve these parameters and to reach a standardized and validated procedure. The results of the Eurohep study and of the French multicentre quality control clearly indicate that optimization and standardization of HCV-RNA PCR techniques are possible and useful to participating laboratories. Indeed, such quality control studies may help PCR laboratories to identify and correct specific failures in their own procedure. Our working group has chosen to preserve this work strategy and has decided to perform each year a quality control of the PCR procedure of each participating laboratory. Furthermore, our group will undertake in the future a new multicentre quality control of the different HCV techniques of molecular biology, including RNA quantification, genotyping and serotyping.

References

1. Choo QL, Kuo G, Weiner AJ, Overby LR, Bradley DW, Houghton M. Isolation of a cDNA clone derived from a blood born non-A, non-B viral hepatitis genome. Science 1989 ; 244 : 359-61.
2. Kuo G, Choo QL, Alter HJ, et al. An assay for circulating antibodies to a major etiologic virus of human non-A, non-B hepatitis. Science 1989 ; 244 : 362-364.
3. Saiki RK, Scharf S, Faloona F, et al. Enzymatic amplification of β-globin genomic sequences and restriction site analysis for diagnosis of sickle cell anemia. Science 1985 ; 230 : 1350-4.
4. Wiener AJ, Kuo G, Bradley DW, et al. Detection of hepatitis C viral sequences in non-A, non-B hepatitis. Lancet 1990 ; 335 : 1-3.
5. Garson JA, Tedder RS, Briggs M, et al. Detection of hepatitis C viral sequences in blood donations by « nested » polymerase chain reaction and prediction of infectivity. Lancet 1990 ; 335 : 1419-22.
6. Shimizu YK, Weiner AJ, Rosenblatt J, et al. Early events in hepatitis C virus infection of chimpanzees. Proc Natl Acad Sci USA 1990 ; 87 : 6441-4.
7. Alberti A, Chemello L, Cavalleto D, et al. Antibody to hepatitis C virus and liver disease in volunteer blood donors. Ann Intern Med 1991 ; 114 : 1010-2.
8. Kanai K, Iwata J, Nakao K, Kako M, Okamoto H. Suppression of hepatitis C virus RNA by interferon alpha. Lancet 1990 ; 336 : 245.
9. Thaler MM, Park CK, Landers DV, et al. Vertical transmission of hepatitis C virus. Lancet 1991 ; 338 : 17-8.
10. Roudot-Thoraval F, Pawlotsky JM, Thiers V, et al. Lack of mother-to-infant transmission of hepatitis C virus in human immunodeficiency virus-seronegative women : a prospective study with hepatitis C virus RNA testing. Hepatology 1993 ; 17 : 772-7.
11. Wu DY, Ugozzoli L, Pal BK, Qian J, Wallace RB. The effect of temperature and oligonucleotide primer length on the specificity and efficiency of amplification by the polymerase chain reaction. Cell Biol 1991 ; 10 : 233-7.
12. Castillo I, Bartolome J, Quiroga JA, Carreno V. Comparison of several PCR procedures for detection of serum HCV-RNA using different regions of the HCV genome. J Virol Methods 1992 ; 38 : 71-80.
13. Bukh J, Purcell RH, Miller RH. Importance of primer selection for the detection of hepatitis C virus RNA with the polymerase chain reaction assay. Proc Natl Acad Sci USA 1992 ; 89 : 187-91.
14. Chomczynski P, Sacchi N. Single step method of RNA isolation by acid guanidinium thiocyanate phenol chloroform extraction. Anal Biochem 1987 ; 62 : 156-9.
15. Kwok S, Higuchi R. Avoiding false-positives with PCR. Nature 1989 ; 339 : 237-8.
16. Zaaijer HL, Cuypers HTM, Reesink HW, Winkel IN, Gerken G, Lelie PN. Reliability of polymerase chain reaction for detection of hepatitis C virus. Lancet 1993 ; 341 : 722-4.
17. French Study Group for the Standardization of Hepatitis C virus Polymerase Chain Reaction. Improvement of hepatitis C virus RNA polymerase chain reaction through a multicentre quality control study. J Virol Methods, in press.
18. Willems M, Moshage H, Nevens F, Fevery J, Yap SH. Plasma collected from heparinized blood is not suitable for HCV-RNA detection by conventional RT-PCR assay. J Virol Methods 1993 ; 42 : 127-30.
19. Lau JYN, Davis GL, Kniffen J, et al. Significance of serum hepatitis C virus RNA levels in chronic hepatitis C. Lancet 1993 ; 341 : 1501-4.

6

Branched DNA (bDNA) quantitation of hepatitis C viral RNA in patient sera

J. KOLBERG, R. SANCHÉZ-PESCADOR, J. DETMER, M. COLLINS, P. SHERIDAN, P. NEUWALD, J. WILBER, P. DAILEY, M. URDEA

Chiron Corporation, Emeryville, CA, USA.

HCV RNA detection has been widely applied to the study and clinical management of chronic hepatitis infection. In patients or blood donors with indeterminate serology results, HCV RNA detection has been used to determine infectivity. Semi-quantitative, and more recently, quantitative, detection has been used to identify candidates for interferon (IFN) therapy and to monitor viral load during the course of chronic infection and antiviral treatment [1].

Target and signal amplification methods have been used in the detection and quantitation of HCV RNA. Whereas the target amplification method, polymerase chain reaction (PCR), has been successfully employed by many groups for the detection of HCV RNA, it is at best semi-quantitative. In contrast, branched DNA (bDNA) signal amplification is a highly precise, accurate and simple method for HCV RNA quantitation.

The bDNA method uses a solution-phase sandwich assay format (see Figure 1). A crude proteinase K lysate of RNA or DNA is denatured and hybridized in solution to two sets of oligonucleotide target probes to mediate capture and to bind bDNA amplifiers. These approximately 50-base fragments contain a portion that is complementary to the target (20-40 bases) and a second portion (20 bases) that is used to capture the probe-target complex onto an oligonucleotide modified microwell or to bind the bDNA to the probe-target fragment and labe-

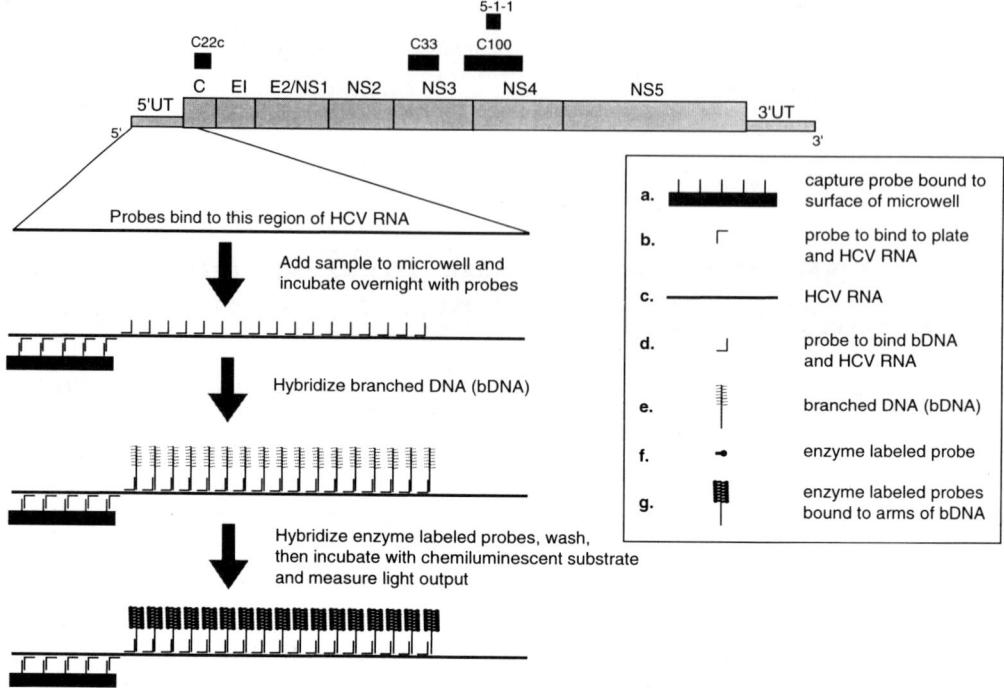

Figure 1. Diagrammatic representation of the HCV genome and the bDNA assay procedure.

led probes. Several of each type (5-50) can be used. Once the probe-target complex is bound to the microwell, the well is washed. The bDNA is then hybridized. After a wash, the bDNA is labeled with an alkaline phosphatase probe (18 bases). Finally, the complex is detected and quantified with a dioxetane substrate that can be triggered by an enzyme, yielding a chemiluminescent output detectable with a luminometer.

The method has been applied to the detection of CMV, HBV, HCV, and HIV [2]. Between 50 and 1,000 µl of serum or plasma or cells in buffer is used for the assays. DNA assays (CMV and HBV) require a denaturation step with NaOH. Cutoff values of between 3,000 and 20,000 molecules per well (based on negative population studies) are used for the assays. For HCV RNA quantitation, a sample of 50 µl of serum is employed.

Target probes for the HCV RNA quantitation assay (Quantiplex™ HCV-RNA) are based on sequences of the highly conserved 5' portion of the genome. The probes cover the untranslated region and part of the core gene. Because the probes are from a highly conserved region [3], clinical samples which represent different genotypes are clearly detected by the bDNA assay (Table I) even though they were not detected by the first generation EIA. To test the accuracy of quantitation of the bDNA assay, carefully quantitated « in vitro » transcripts representing subtype 1b and subtype 3a [4] were prepared. These transcripts were tested in the bDNA assay and the quantitation of the two transcripts were compared. The signal ratio of subtype 1b/subtype 3a was 1.6 [5].

Table I. Comparison of Immunoassays and RNA Detection.

Specimen	Subtype (4)	EIA-1*	EIA-2*	RIBA*	RT-PCR 5'UT	RT-PCR E1	RT-PCR NS5	Chiron Quantiplex™ HCV RNA
GH77918	1b	NR	R	I	+	+	+	+
GJ61353	1b	NR	R	R	+	+	+	+
GC16799	2b	NR	R	R	+	−	+	+
LX91250	2b	NR	R	R	+	−	+	+
LQ41461	2b	NR	R	R	+	−	+	+
FC71921	2b	NR	R	R	+	−	+	+
GJ61329	3a	NR	R	I	+	+	+	+
S21	3a	NR	R	I	+	+	+	+

* NR = Non-reactive   R = Reactive   I = Indeterminate

The limit of detection of the bDNA assay was set at 350,000 equivalents per milliliter (Eq/ml) based upon an analysis of HCV positive and negative specimens. The reported clinical sensitivity of the bDNA assay ranges from 72 %-95 % depending upon the patient population [1, 6]. We are currently developing an improved assay which will have increased sensitivity. In patients with HCV-associated chronic hepatitis, chronic active hepatitis, chronic persistent hepatitis, and cirrhosis, HCV RNA levels range from undetectable (by any technique) to more than 1×10^8 HCV Eq/ml.

In Figure 2, the reproducibility of the bDNA assay is demonstrated. Four separate patient samples (the four panels) were tested by two operators on three days with five microwell plates. As can be seen from the error bars, less than a three-fold variation in the viral load was consistently obtained.

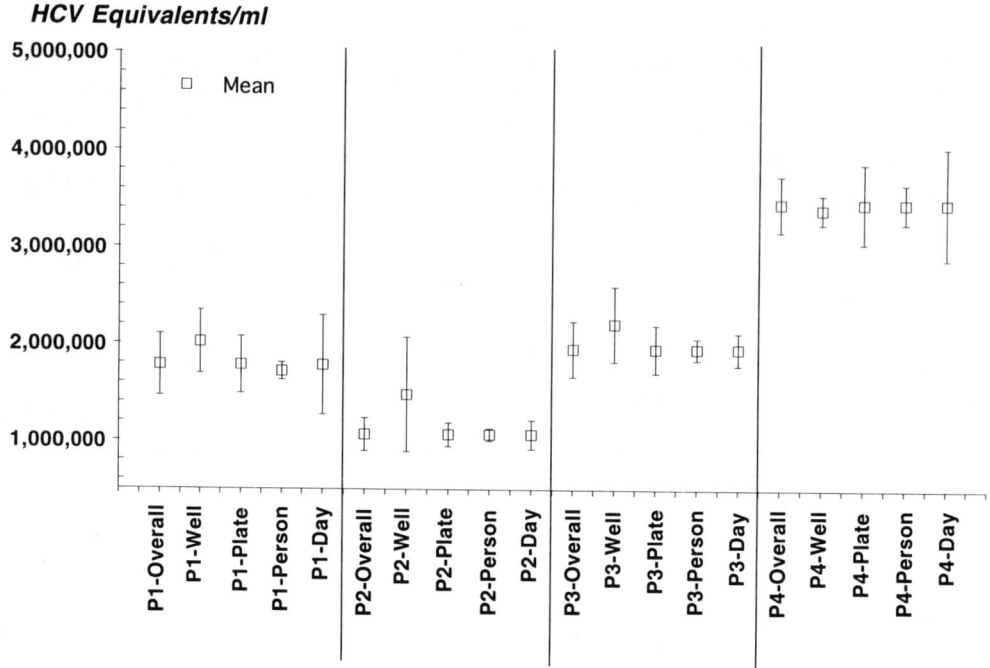

Figure 2. Data for this experiment were generated by testing four HCV positive sera (P1, P2, P3, P4) in quadruplicate in each of two plates by two operators on three consecutive days. In total, data from twelve plates are presented.

Processing and storage conditions can significantly influence the level of HCV RNA in patient specimens. There is a progressive loss in HCV RNA reactivity when the time from clot formation until centrifugation exceeds two hours. Davis et al. [7] found a 25 % loss in reactivity after six hours and a 44 % loss after 24 hours. No loss of HCV RNA activity has been observed after three freeze-thaw cycles.

It is generally presumed that HCV RNA can always be found in the serum of patients with chronic hepatitis patients. However, this is not always the case. Wide fluctuations in HCV RNA have been reported, with levels sometimes falling below detection limits of bDNA and PCR assays. The reasons for these fluctuations are not understood.

In acute infection, HCV RNA is usually detectable at least 40 days before serum ALT levels. Following the early peak, at levels exceeding $10^{7.5}$ HCV Eq/ml, RNA levels tend to fall to lower levels within about 10 weeks with seroconversion (Figure 3).

Patients with chronic HCV infection show fluctuating levels of both

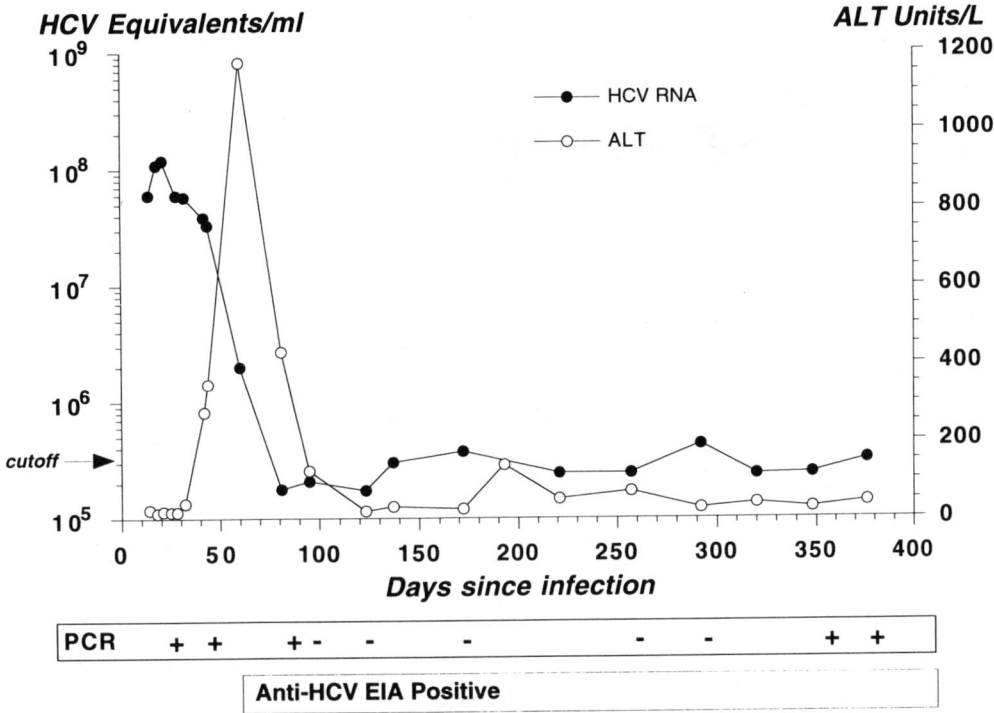

Figure 3. Patient was transfused on day 0. Levels of HCV-RNA, ALT and Anti-HCV antibodies were monitored for over a year post-transfusion.

HCV RNA and ALT over time. In some patients, changes in HCV RNA levels tend to precede ALT spikes. In others, there is no clear pattern of correspondence between the two markers. Whereas HCV RNA can fluctuate by over a million-fold, ALT levels vary by no more than 45-fold (from normal, 35 U/L, up to 1500 U/L).

In Figure 4, the HCV-RNA levels of three chronic hepatitis C patients on IFN therapy are shown. Figure 4a shows a « typical » responder and Figure 4b shows a « typical » nonresponder. Figure 4c shows a patient with an apparent response in ALT, but raising levels of RNA. Response to IFN therapy is based on normalization of ALT levels for at least one year following the end of therapy.

During and after IFN therapy, the timing and frequency of ALT and RNA determinations may be critical in identifying trends towards response, virologic relapse, and/or biochemical relapse. For example, patients who show a biochemical response to IFN therapy (*i.e.* normalization of ALT) have not necessarily cleared detectable virus from

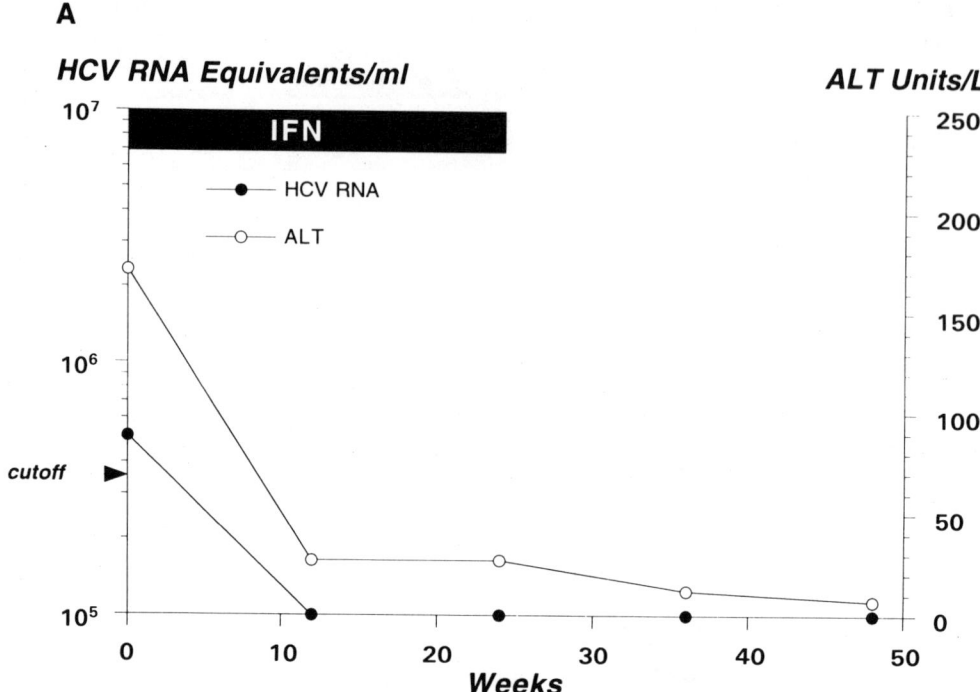

Figure 4. Data from three chronic hepatitis C patients on IFN therapy is presented. Patients were given 360 MU of natural IFNα for and followed for six to twelve months. (A) Data from a patient classified as a responder. ALT values are normalized for at least one year following the end of therapy. HCV-RNA is undetectable by both the bDNA assay and RT-PCR, (B) Data from a patient classified as a non-responder. Both ALT and HCV RNA levels drop during IFN therapy but return quickly after the end of therapy, and (C) Data from a patient in which ALT values decrease to near normal level, but RNA levels continue to rise.

their blood, making them susceptible to virologic relapse (Figure 4c) [8]. In some cases, viremia disappears and then returns ; in other cases, it remains at pretreatment levels. In contrast, biochemical non-responders can lose detectable virus, temporarily or long-term. Quantitating HCV RNA in the liver and peripheral blood mononuclear cells, which are known to be an extrahepatic reservoir for the virus, may also help to predict and evaluate response to IFN therapy.

Bhandari and co-workers [9] have shown that the distributions of HCV RNA and histologic features are consistent throughout different parts of the liver. We have quantitated HCV RNA in biopsy specimens from both the right and left lobes of the liver and also found

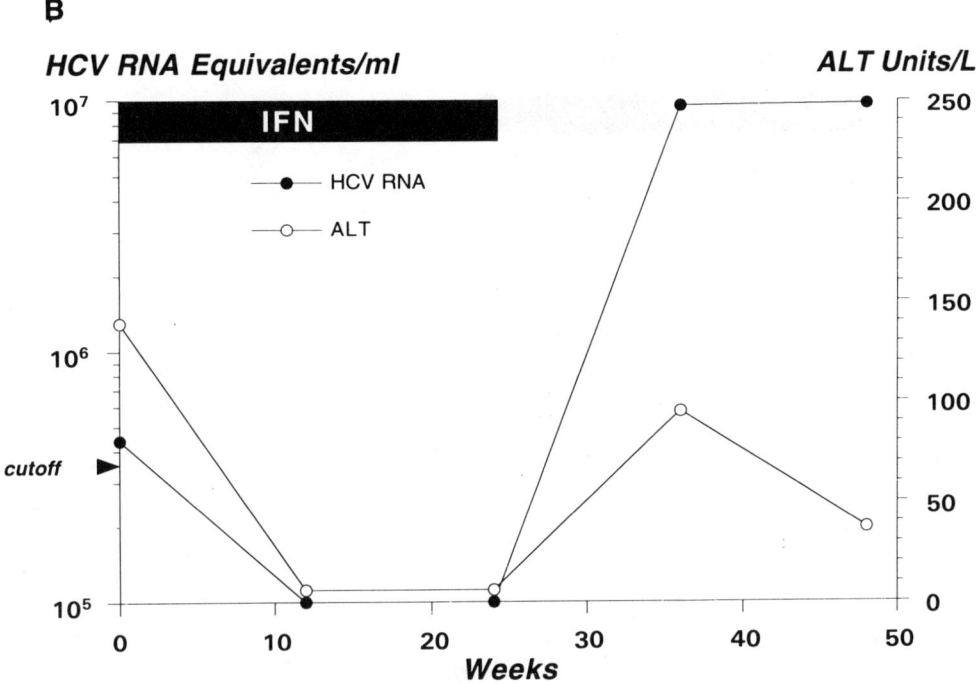

no differences in hepatic HCV RNA distribution [10]. Random needle biopsy can thus be used for obtaining samples for histologic examination and HCV RNA quantitation.

Using the bDNA assay to measure RNA in paired liver and serum specimens from patients with chronic active hepatitis, we found that serum levels reflect those in the liver. The mean ratio of liver to serum HCV RNA levels was 36 (range : 1-138). Patients with chronic persistent hepatitis had lower HCV RNA levels in serum and liver than those with more severe disease [11].

We have analyzed nucleotide sequences of a region of NS5 in HCV samples obtained from throughout the world and have proposed as systematic nomenclature for genotypes based on this analysis [12]. A segment of the NS5 region was used for this analysis because of the availability of PCR primers which efficiently amplify this region and the degree of sequence variation is sufficient for differentiation of genotypes. There is also considerable sequence information available on the 5' untranslated (UT) region, but the sequence homology is quite

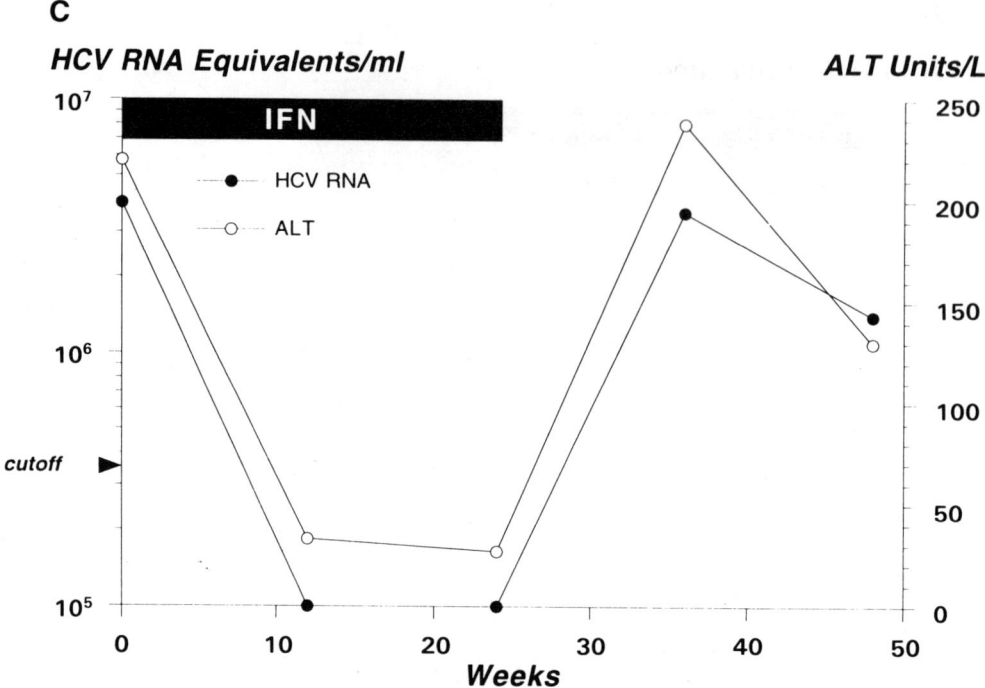

high (> 90 %) making identification of distinct genotypes difficult. In our analysis, 76 sequences in the NS5 region were used [4]. The analysis included 35 sequences previously reported, as well as new sequences not previously reported from samples obtained throughout the world including South America, Africa and the Middle East. Based on phylogenetic analysis of these NS5 sequences, six distinct types could be identified and observed in a phylogenetic tree (Figure 5). Additional sequence variation within types 1, 2 and 3 allows for the classification of distinct subtypes. Phylogenetic analysis provides information on the evolutionary relationship between sequences but is computationally intensive. Simple pair-wise comparison of sequence similarity was also used to compare sequences of NS5. This analysis provided the same classification of type and subtype. The sequence similarity between types is 56 %-72 %. Between subtype the sequence similarity is 74 %-86 % and within a subtype the sequence similarity is > 88 %. A summary of the proposed classification is included (Table II). Sequence analysis of other regions provides the same classification, however the level of sequence similarity differs. Using sequences in 5'UT region where the sequence is quite well conserved, does not allow differentiation of HCV subtypes. Also, sequences which are classified as a particular type based on the NS5 sequence are also classified as

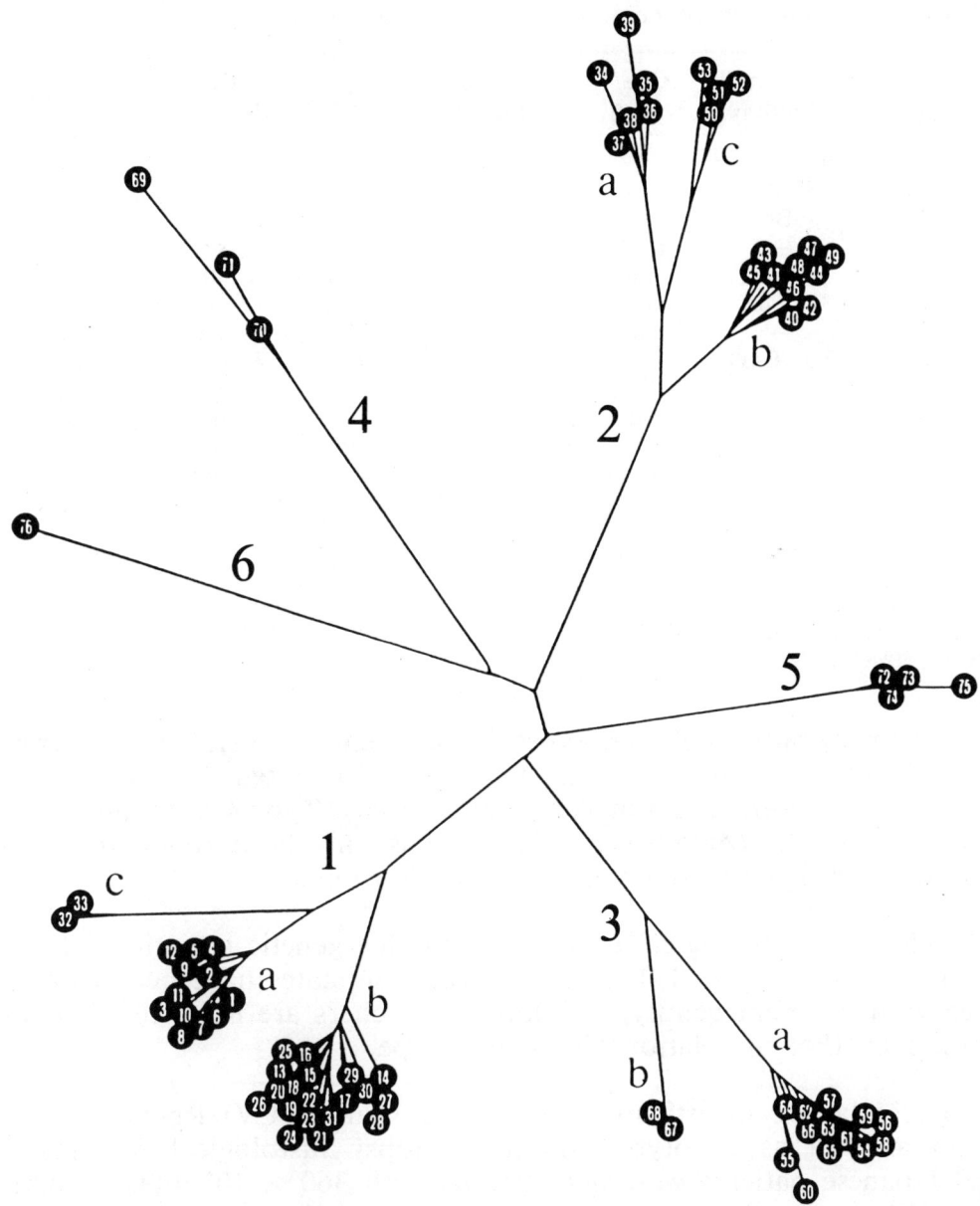

Figure 5. Phylogenetic analysis of NS5 sequences of 76 isolates of HCV, showing six major HCV types and subsidiary grouping within some HCV types; from Simmonds et al. [4].

the same type when other regions are analyzed. It thus appears that the genotype of a sample is the same throughout the entire genome.

Table II. Comparison of nomenclature for HCV types.

Proposed name	Published Example	Cha/ Urdea[1]	Chan/ Simmonds[2]	Enomoto[3]	Mori/ Okamoto[4]	Kohara[5]
1a	HCV-1, -H	I	1a	K-PT	I	nc
1b	HCV-J, -BK	II	1b	K-1	II	I
1c	—	nc*	nc	nc	nc	nc
2a	HC-J6	III	2a	K-2a	III	II
2b	HC-J8	III	2b	K-2b	IV	II
2c	—	III	nc	nc	nc	nc
3a	Ta, E-b1	IV	3	nc	V	nc
3b	Tb	IV	nc	nc	VI	nc
4a	—	nc	4	nc	nc	nc
5a	—	V	nc	nc	nc	nc
6a	—	nc	nc	nc	nc	nc

* not classified

1. Cha et al. [3]
2. Chan et al. [15], Simmonds et al. [16]
3. Enomoto et al. [17]
4. Okamoto et al., Mori et al. [8]
5. Kohara et al. [19]

The distribution of genotypes is different in different countries. Type 1, 2 and 3 are found to be widely distributed. Types 4, 5 and 6 have each been found in very limited areas. Type 4 is found predominantly in the Middle East. Type 5 has only been found in South Africa and Type 6 found only in Hong Kong.

What is the biological importance of this genetic variation ? Some reports have proposed that different disease states have been associated with different genotypes. Many researchers are now studying responce to IFN in relationship to genotype.

Recently, we investigated hepatitis C virus (HCV) RNA quantitation as well as genotype and liver biopsy histological features in 60 Japanese patients who were treated with 360×10^6 units of natural IFN-α for 36 to 48 weeks and were followed for more than 12 months [13]. By using the bDNA assay to measure HCV-RNA levels, all responders had less than 2×10^6 Eq/ml prior to administration of IFN. Of 39 patients with initial RNA levels less than 2×10^6 Eq/ml, 23 (59.0 %) were responders (Figure 6). The genotype was determined for each patient using type specific PCR primers as reported by Okamoto [14]. There was a significant difference

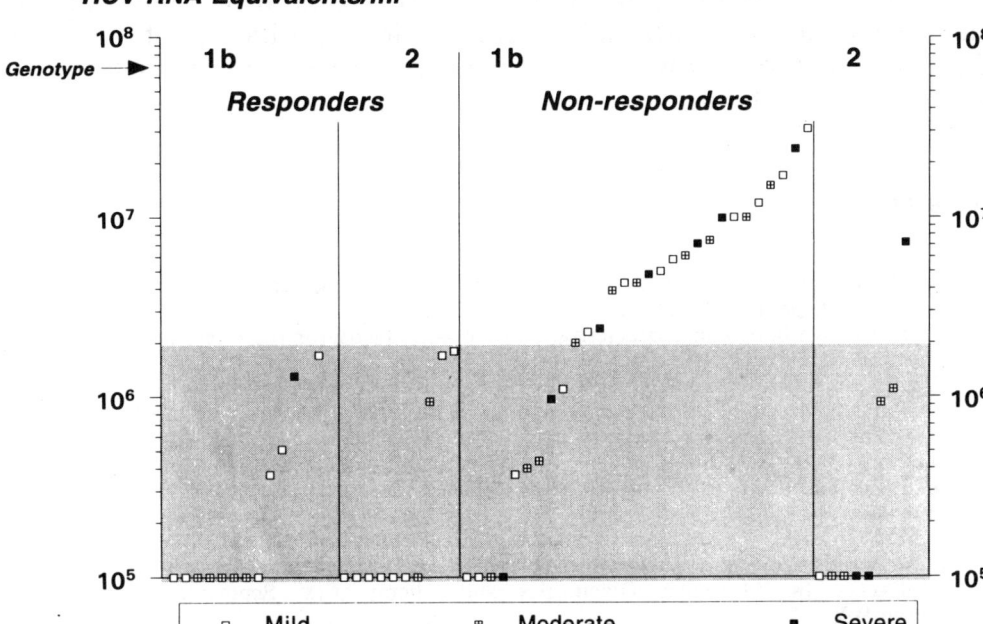

Figure 6. Initial HCV RNA levels of 60 patients treated with 360 MU natural IFN-α and subsequent response to IFN therapy. Genotype was determined by type specific PCR primers [14] and liver histology was classified as mild, moderate or severe chronic hepatitis. All responders had initial HCV RNA levels of less than 2×10^6 Eq/ml.

in RNA levels between subtype 1b and type 2 (2a and 2b) (p < 0.0002). The response to IFN in patients with HCV-RNA subtype levels less than 2×10^6 Eq/ml is independent of genotype. In a multivariate analysis, RNA level was the most statistically significant factor affecting response to IFN. Histologic features were determined for each patient and IFN was ineffective in all patients with initial levels of HCV-RNA greater than 2×10^6 Eq/ml regardless of histologic features. However, in patients with less than 2×10^6 Eq/ml there was a difference in response to IFN between mild and severe chronic hepatitis.

The observation that some genotypes respond more favorably to IFN treatment may be due to the lower average viremia of the better responding genotypes. This needs to be studied more extensively in other patient populations and in additional genotypes. The bDNA assay, which is highly reproducible, and accurately quantitates HCV-RNA levels independent of genotype may be very useful to determine which patients are most likely to respond to IFN treatment. Some researchers have noted significant differences in quantitation of HCV by PCR vs. bDNA ; however, the genotype variation of PCR based methods has not been established.

References

1. Lau JYN, Davis GL, Kniffen J, et al. Significance of serum hepatitis C virus RNA levels in chronic hepatitis C. Lancet 1993 ; 341 : 1501-4.
2. Urdea M. Synthesis and characterization of branch DNA for the direct and quantitative detection of CMV, HBV, HCV and HIV. Clinical Chemistry 1993 ; 39 : 725-6.
3. Cha TA, Beall E, Irvine B, Kolberg J, Chien D, Kuo G, Urdea MS. At least five related, but distinct, hepatitis C viral genotypes exist. Proc Natl Acad Sci USA 1992 ; 89 : 7144-88.
4. Simmonds P, Holmes EC, Cha TA, et al. Classification of hepatitis C virus into six major genotypes and a series of subtypes by phylogenetic tree analysis. J Gen Virol 1993 ; 74 : 2391-9.
5. Collins M, Lagier R, Sanchéz-Pescador R, et al. Preparation of gold standard HCV type 1 and 3 RNAs and quantitation using branched DNA signal amplification. (Abstr.) ASM Conference on Molecular Diagnostics and Therapeutics, September 26-30, 1993, Moran WY.
6. Yuki N, Hayashi N, Kamada T. HCV viraemia and liver injury in symptom-free blood donors. Lancet 1993 ; 342 : 444.
7. Davis GL, Lau JYN, Urdea MS, Neuwald PD, Wilber JC, Lindsay K, Perrillo RP, Albrecht J. Quantitative detection of hepatitis C virus (HCV) RNA by a solid-phase signal amplification method : definition of optimal conditions for specimen collection and clinical applications in interferon-treated patients. 1994, in press.
8. Shindo M, DiBisceglie AM, Cheung L, Shih JWK, Cristiano K, Feinstone SM, Hoofnagle JH. Decrease in serum hepatitis C viral RNA during alpha interferon therapy for chronic hepatitis C. Ann Intern Med 1991 ; 9 : 700-4.
9. Bhandari BN, Dailey PJ, Ferrell L, Bacchei P, Wright L. HCV RNA level and histopathology is similar in needle biopsy from different parts of the liver. (Abstr.) Digestive Diseases Meeting, May 15-18 1994, New Orleans, LA.
10. Idrovo V, Jeffers L, Coelho-Little E, et al. HCV-RNA quantitation in right and left lobes of the liver in patients with chronic hepatitis C. Chiron Corporation, Emeryville, CA and University of Miami School of Medicine and VAMC, Miami, FL.
11. Coelho-Little ME, Jeffers LJ, Reddy R, Schiff ER, Dailey P. Correlation of HCV-RNA quantitation in serum and liver tissue of patients with chronic hepatitis C. 1994, submitted.
12. Simmonds P, Alberti A, Alter HJ, et al. A proposed system for nomenclature of genotypes for hepatitis C virus. Hepatology 1994 (in press).
13. Yamada G, Takatani M, Fumitoshi K, et al. Efficacy of interferon-α therapy in chronic hepatitis C depends primarily on HCV RNA level. Submitted, 1994.
14. Okamoto M, Sugiyama Y, Okada S, Kurai K, Akahane Y, Sugai Y, Tanaka T. Typing hepatitis C virus by polymerase chain reaction with type-specific primers : application to clinical surveys and tracing infection sources. J Gen Virol 1992 ; 73 : 673-9.
15. Chan SW, McOmish F, Holmes EC, et al. Analysis of a new hepatitis C virus type and its phylogenetic relationship of existing variants. J Gen Virol 1992 ; 73 : 1131-41.
16. Simmonds P, McOmish F, Yap PL, et al. Sequence variability in the 5' non-coding region of hepatitis C virus : identification of a new virus type and restrictions on sequence diversity. J Gen Virol 1993 ; 74 : 661-8.
17. Enomoto N, Takada A, Nakao T, Date T. There are two major types of hepatitis C virus in Japan. Biochem Biophys Res Commun 1990 ; 170 : 1021-25.

18. Mori S, Kato N, Yagyu A, *et al.* A new type of hepatitis C virus in patients in Thailand. Biochem Biophys Res Commun 1992 ; 183 : 334-42.
19. Kohara KT, Kohara M, Yamaguchi K, *et al.* A second group of hepatitis C viruses. Virus Genes 1991 ; 5 : 243-54.

7

Specific detection of HCV RNA using NASBA™ as a diagnostic tool

P. SILLEKENS[1], W. KOK[1], B. VAN GEMEN[1], P. LENS[1], H. HUISMAN[2], Th. CUYPERS[2], T. KIEVITS[1]

[1] Organon Teknika, Boseind 15, 5280 AB Boxtel, The Netherlands;
[2] Central Laboratory of the Netherlands Red Cross Blood Transfusion Service, Plesmanlaan 125, 1066 CX Amsterdam, The Netherlands.

Introduction

Soon after the introduction of serologic screening for hepatitis B virus (HBV) in blood donors, it became clear that not all cases of transfusion-associated hepatitis could be explained by infection with this virus. It appeared that another virus, now known as the hepatitis C virus (HCV), is the etiological agent of most of these posttransfusion non-A, non-B (NANB) hepatitis cases [1, 2]. The nucleic acid sequence of this single-stranded RNA virus was determined from cDNA clones derived from the nucleic acid extracts of the plasma of an experimentally infected chimpanzee [1]. This provided the basis for the construction of recombinant peptides representing putative HCV proteins [2]. Cloned HCV peptides were employed in anti-HCV enzyme immunoassays and now serological testing to detect antibodies to HCV in blood donors is the principal measure to prevent post-transfusion NANB hepatitis. However, in the absence of tissue culture of the virus, electron microscopy or assays for viral antigen, the direct detection of HCV is by necessity dependent upon nucleic acid hybridization methods. Of the available methods, amplification of HCV RNA commends itself by virtue of the extreme sensitivity and consequent ability to detect the often very low levels of HCV RNA that are present in clinical samples. An amplification technology that directly uses RNA as its target (NASBA™) and its application in qualitative and quantitative assays for detection of HCV RNA are described.

Principle of the NASBA™ amplification technique

Nucleic acid amplification techniques have been employed for detection of many classes of infectious agents including a wide range of viruses [3]. Especially for viruses causing latent infections or infections in which antigen production is limited or in which serological responses are delayed or even absent, amplification techniques have proved useful for diagnosis. Also in case of an HCV infection, direct detection of the virus as a marker for an actual ongoing infection can only be achieved by amplification of HCV RNA due to the fact that the virus titer frequently is low [4-6]. Since HCV is an RNA virus and DNA is the substrate for most amplification technologies, the RNA first has to be reverse-transcribed to cDNA which subsequently can be amplified. However, the principal target of NASBA™ is RNA [7, 8], enabling direct amplification of HCV genome sequences without the need of a preceding reverse transcription step. Using a natural RNA template, a standard NASBA™ reaction comprises three enzymes, two specific primers, nucleoside triphosphates, and appropriate buffer components. The three enzymes involved are T7 RNA polymerase, avian myeloblastosis virus (AMV) reverse transcriptase, and RNase H, each acting continuously on its appropriate substrate(s). Following a single RNA template molecule through the NASBA™ process illustrates how amplification of the target RNA is achieved by the concerted action of these three enzymes. The reaction starts with hybridization of an oligonucleotide primer that contains a T7 RNA polymerase binding site to the target RNA. Reverse transcriptase elongates the primer, creating a cDNA copy of the RNA template and forming an RNA/DNA hybrid. RNase H recognizes this hybrid as substrate and hydrolyses the RNA portion of the hybrid leaving single-stranded DNA. A second oligonucleotide primer anneals to the new DNA strand again forming a substrate suitable for reverse transcriptase extension. This extension finally renders the promoter portion of the nucleic acid sequence double-stranded and transcriptionally active. Recognizing the now functional promoter, T7 RNA polymerase produces multiple copies of antisense RNA transcripts of the original target sequence. Each new antisense RNA molecule can in its turn again be converted to a T7 promoter containing double-stranded cDNA in a similar way, except that primer annealing and extension occur in reverse order because the newly generated RNA template is opposite in orientation to the original target. Again many copies are generated from each RNA target that re-enters the reaction resulting in exponential amplification. The NASBA™ reaction continues in a self-sustained manner under isothermal conditions achieving dramatic amplification in a short period of time. Amplification of approximately 10^6-10^9 fold is obtained within 90 minutes.

NASBA™ for detection of HCV RNA

Prior to amplification, HCV RNA has to be purified from plasma, serum, or blood. This can be achieved by acid guanidinium thiocyanate (GuSCN) lysis of the viral particles, followed by adsorption of the nucleic acid to silica [9]. After subsequent washing steps with GuSCN wash buffer [9], ethanol, and acetone, bound nucleic acid is eluted and used for specific amplification in NASBA™ reactions. The method produces viral RNA of adequate quality and has the advantage of eliminating the need for phenol extraction and alcohol precipitation steps.

Following RNA isolation, the reaction for amplification of HCV RNA was set up by mixing all ingredients except the enzymes. The mixture was incubated at 65 °C during 5 min to denature any secondary structure in the RNA. Then a mixture of the three enzymes was added followed by a 90 min incubation at 41 °C. The specificity of the reaction is determined by the two oligonucleotide primers that are specific for the sequence of interest. To circumvent sensitivity problems arising from the observed sequence heterogeneity between different HCV isolates [10-23], NASBA™ primers were derived from the 5'-noncoding region, which is the most highly conserved sequence of the HCV genome [10, 24-26]. However, even within the 5'-noncoding region sequence heterogeneity is observed, but most nucleotide variations appear to be located in domains interspersed with regions of no sequence variation [27]. In order to obtain matching with all HCV types NASBA™ primers were based on two of these conserved regions. A third conserved region could then be used for general detection of amplified HCV RNA of any kind. On the other hand, hybridization of the amplified products to oligonucleotides directed against the variable domains of the 5'-noncoding region that are contained within the amplimer, enables determination of the genotype and subtype of the virus present in a patient specimen [28, 29].

Amplified products of a NASBA™ reaction can in principle be detected on ethidium bromide-stained gels, but often poor resolution of short RNA fragments hampers interpretation of the results. However, since the product of a NASBA™ reaction is single-stranded RNA, it can easily be diagnosed by hybridization with sequence-specific probes. Two methods of detection were performed. Using a ^{32}P-end-labelled oligonucleotide probe, amplification products can be detected after immobilization on Northern blots. Figure 1 shows a typical Northern blot hybridization result for a panel of 10 patient samples that were analyzed for the presence of HCV RNA. Nucleic acid was extracted by the guanidinium salt/silica method [9] and amplified in duplicate together with nucleic acid extracted from two negative control samples (Figure 1, samples 11 and 12). The detection sensitivity of the amplification method, as determined from a 10-fold dilution series of *in vitro* generated target RNA, was about 10-100 HCV viral genome equivalents (Figure 1).

Since radio-active detection has major drawbacks, a non-radio-active hybridization method for identification of NASBA™ products was developed, the so-called enzyme-linked gel assay (ELGA). Again making use of the single-stranded character of the amplimer, horseradish peroxidase-conjugated oligonucleotide probes (HRP-probes) allow for liquid hybridization. Subsequent electrophoresis of the hybridization reaction discriminates between free HRP-probe and HRP-probe that has specifically hybridized to NASBA™ product. The gel retardation assay is followed by direct staining of the HRP in the gel. The detection of HCV RNA in NASBA™ reactions using ELGA is shown in Figure 2. Semi-quantitative analysis of three patient samples and a negative control sample was performed by limited dilution in combination with ELGA. Reactive and non-reactive samples could clearly be distinguished by the position of the HRP signals in the gel.

In the dilution series of the *in vitro* generated target RNA that is shown in Figure 2, the NASBA™ reaction that was spiked with 10^3 molecules did not reveal any specific product. In case of a patient specimen such a negative reaction might wrongly lead to the conclusion that the patient is negative for HCV RNA. Therefore, to discriminate between a falsely negative reaction and a truly non-reactive sample, a system control RNA was introduced. This system control RNA contains the same primer binding sites as the target RNA. However, compared to the wild-type RNA, it contains an additional sequence insert, thereby generating an amplimer of different size and internal sequence.

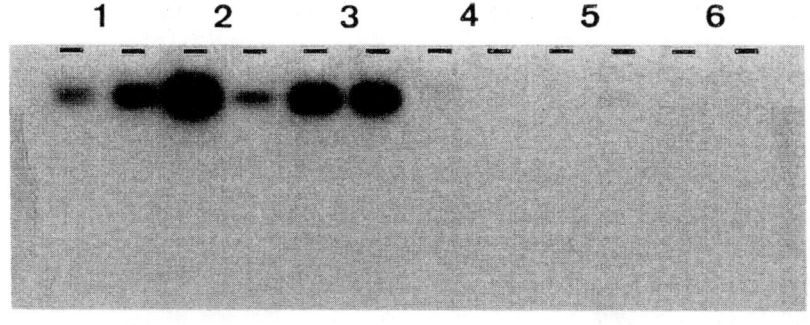

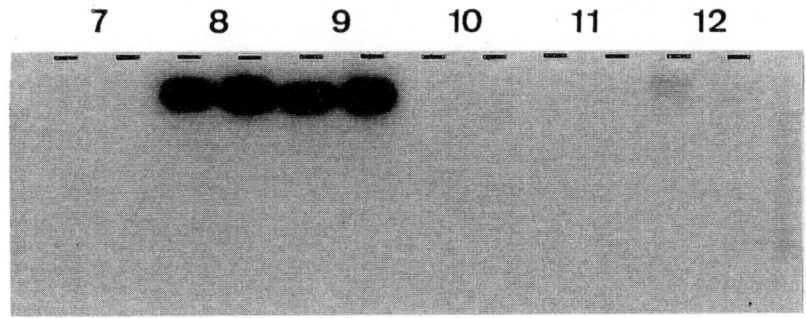

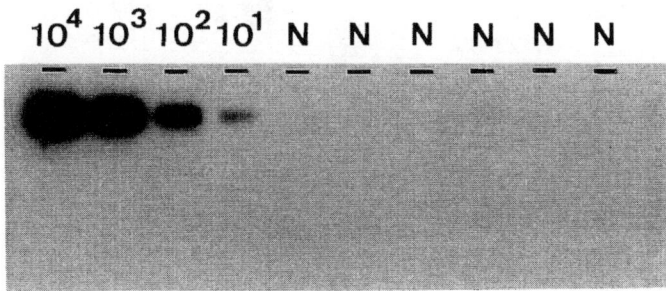

Figure 1. Detection of HCV RNA by Northern blot analysis. Nucleic acid extracted from ten patient plasmas and two negative control plasmas was amplified in duplicate with primers derived from the 5'-noncoding region of the HCV genome. After NASBA™ amplification, reaction products were run on a 1 % agarose gel, transferred to a nylon membrane, and hybridized with a ^{32}P-end-labelled oligonucleotide. Lanes : (1-10) patient plasmas ; (11,12) HCV-negative control plasmas ; (10^4-10^1) 10-fold dilution series of *in vitro* generated input RNA containing 10^4 down to 10 molecules ; (N) no template NASBA™ reactions.

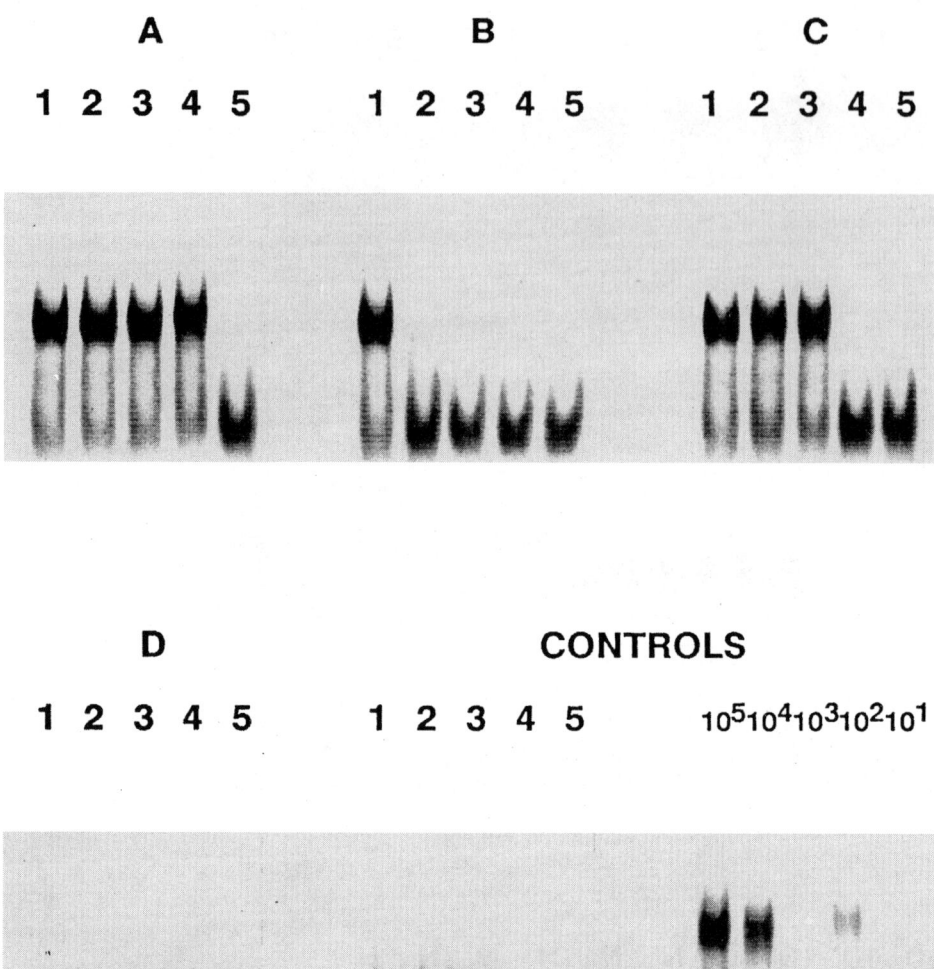

Figure 2. Detection of HCV RNA by ELGA after limited dilution NASBA™ amplification. A 10-fold dilution series of nucleic acid extracted from three patient plasmas (A-C) and a negative control plasma (D) was amplified with primers derived from the 5'-noncoding region of the HCV genome. After NASBA™ amplification, reaction products were hybridized in solution to an HRP-labelled oligonucleotide, run on a 7 % polyacrylamide gel and stained with TMB substrate. Lanes : (1) undiluted nucleic acid extract ; (2-5) 10-fold dilutions of nucleic acid extract ; Controls : (1-5) no template NASBA™ reactions ; (10^5-10^1) 10-fold dilution series of *in vitro* generated RNA containing 10^5 down to 10 molecules of input RNA.

Prior to nucleic acid isolation, the system control RNA is added to each specimen. The consequent system control signal enables detection of falsely negative test results (Figure 3). When no virus RNA is present in a specimen, the NASBA™ system should amplify and detect the spiked system control RNA (Figure 3, lane 3). In case of an HCV RNA positive sample amplification of the wild-type RNA outnumbers the system control RNA (Figure 3, lane 1). Only specimens containing low levels of HCV RNA may occasionally result in a weak signal from the internal control RNA (Figure 3, lane 2). In case neither an internal control signal nor the wild-type signal appears, nucleic acid extraction and/or amplification has (have) failed and the specimen may be falsely non-reactive (Figure 3, lane 4).

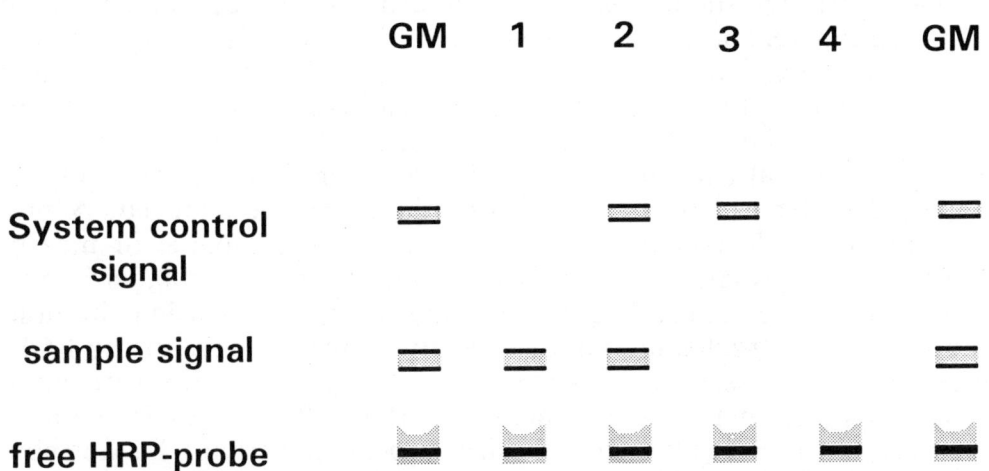

Figure 3. Schematic diagram of the possible gel patterns in ELGA after NASBA™ amplification with system control RNA. Lanes : (GM) gel marker pattern ; (1) positive sample ; (2) weakly positive sample ; (3) negative sample ; (4) NASBA™ failure reaction.

Quantitation of HCV viraemia

To see how serum HCV RNA levels change in relation to the natural evolution of chronic HCV infection, to find out possible correlations between HCV virus titers and clinical indices, or to monitor the effect of antiviral drugs like interferon-α, used to treat patients with chronic HCV infection, all are examples that call for quantitative nucleic acid amplification assays. Several quantitative reverse transcriptase polymerase chain reaction (RT-PCR) methods have been developed. Those include methods based on externally amplified standards [30-32], limited dilution of cDNA [5, 33, 34], or co-amplification of known amounts of competitive mutated templates [6, 35]. Theoretically, competitive amplification of an internal standard is the most accurate way of measuring nucleic acid levels, provided the amplification efficiency of the wild-type and of the internal standard target sequence is equivalent [36, 37]. However, assays based on this principle are very labour intensive, since quantitation is accomplished by addition of a dilution series of the competitor molecule to a set of reactions containing a constant amount of nucleic acid extracted from the specimen to be quantitated. Consequently multiple amplification reactions per sample are needed to quantify a certain target. In theory, the number of amplifications could be reduced to just one if several mutually distinguishable internal standards would be spiked to an amplification reaction instead of one. Based on the assumption that each of the competitor molecules in the reaction is amplified with equal efficiency and to the same extent as the wild-type sequence, a calibration curve can be calculated from the internal standards. From this curve the original concentration of the target molecule in the sample, amplified under exactly the same conditions, can be deduced. A prerequisite for such a method is a detection system capable of measuring the ratios of wild-type nucleic acid and the internal standards over a broad dynamic range. These conditions were met in using the non-radio-active electrochemiluminescence (ECL) technology. In the ECL-based detection assay an oligonucleotide labelled with the ruthenium chelate tris-[2,2'-bypiridine]-ruthenium (II) (TBR) is used in a liquid hybridization format [38]. The physical process underlying ECL is characterized by light emission. The emission of photons is generated from the TBR complex by chemical reactions initiated by an applied voltage.

A quantitative NASBA™ (Q-NASBA™) assay for HCV RNA was developed in which three competitor RNAs (Q-RNAs) were spiked as internal standards to an HCV RNA positive sample. The Q-RNAs differed from the wild-type target sequence only by a randomization of 20 nucleotides. This prevented differences in amplification efficiency due to the length of the amplified product. Amplified wild-type and Q-RNAs could be distinguished by hybridization with ECL-probes complementary to the wild-type sequence or each of the randomized sequences in the Q-RNAs. Feasibility of this one-tube HCV RNA Q-NASBA™ assay was demonstrated by quantitation of known amounts of *in vitro* generated target RNA. A typical result is shown in Figure 4. An amount of 10^3 *in vitro* generated wild-type HCV

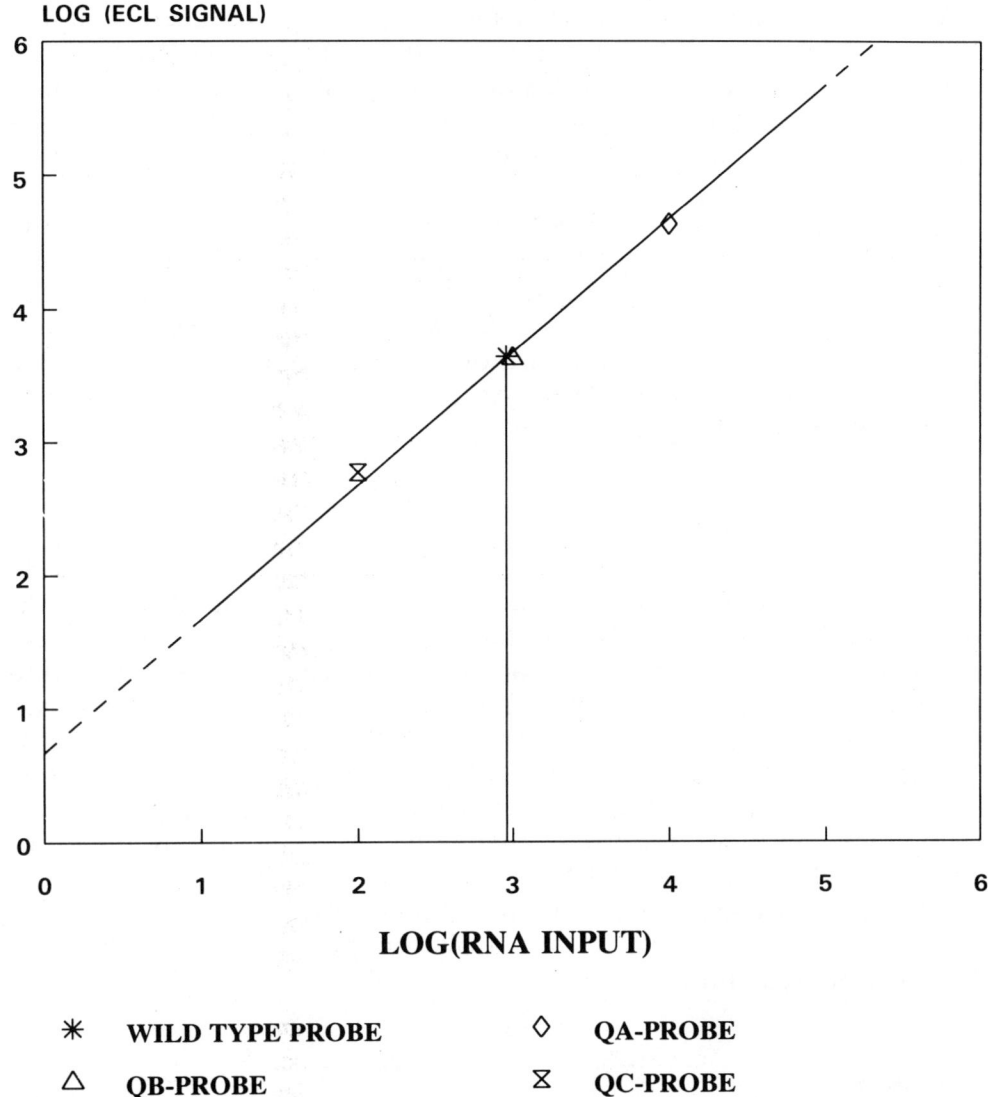

* WILD TYPE PROBE ◇ QA-PROBE
△ QB-PROBE ⌛ QC-PROBE

Figure 4. Quantitation of in vitro generated target RNA with the one tube HCV RNA Q-NASBA™. 10^3 molecules of *in vitro* RNA were amplified in the presence of 10^4 molecules of Qa-RNA, 10^3 molecules of Qb-RNA, and 10^2 molecules of Qc-RNA. Amplified products were analyzed with ECL-labelled oligonucleotide probes specific for wild-type RNA and each of the competitor Q-RNAs. The log of the ECL-signal of the competitor products is graphed as a function of the log of the known amounts of each competitor RNA added. The log of the initial amount of sample RNA can be derived from the ECL-signal for wild-type RNA.

RNA molecules was mixed with 10^4 Qa-RNA molecules, 10^3 Qb-RNA molecules, and 10^2 Qc-RNA molecules and subsequently amplified in a single NASBA™ reaction. Equal amounts of the reaction were aliquoted over four tubes and in each tube amplified products were captured onto paramagnetic beads by hybridization to an oligonucleotide immobilized on the beads itself by a biotin-avidin interaction. Simultaneous hybridization to one of the ECL-labelled probes, specific for either wild-type RNA or one of the Q-RNAs, and subsequent ECL-analysis allowed for calculation of the initial input of wild-type RNA. The result of the quantitation shown in Figure 4 was $10^{2.95}$ molecules of wild-type input RNA. Different concentrations of input RNA revealed that quantitation by extrapolation to 1.0 log beyond the amounts of the Q-RNAs added, still gave reliable results and that reproducibility of the assay was within 0.5 log.

In conclusion, the one-tube quantitation NASBA™ assay for HCV RNA is much less labour intensive due to reduction of the number of amplifications to just one, whereas the reliability and accuracy of the method are comparable to those of previously developed NASBA™ quantitation methods employing multiple amplifications per specimen [39, 40]. An additional advantage of this one-tube quantitative protocol is that the Q-RNAs can be added to the specimen prior to nucleic acid isolation. Provided the Q-RNAs are extracted with the same efficiency as the wild-type RNA, the effect of any possible loss of nucleic acid during isolation, which might dramatically influence the outcome of quantitation, is ruled out. As only the initial ratios of wild-type RNA to the Q-RNAs are used to deduce the amount of input wild-type RNA, in this method quantitation is not effected by the efficiency of the nucleic acid isolation procedure preceding the amplification reaction.

References

1. Choo QL, Kuo G, Weiner AJ, et al. Isolation of a cDNA clone derived from a blood-borne non-A, non-B viral hepatitis genome. Science 1989 ; 244 : 359-62.
2. Kuo G, Choo QL, Alter HJ, et al. An assay for circulating antibodies to a major etiologic virus of human non-A, non-B hepatitis. Science 1989 ; 244 : 362-4.
3. Kwok S and Sninsky JJ. In : PCR Technology, edited by Erlich, H.A. Stockton Press, 1989.
4. Hsu HH, Wright TL, Luba D, et al. Failure to detect hepatitis C virus genome in human secretions with the polymerase chain reaction. Hepatology 1991 ; 14 : 763-7.
5. Simmonds P, Zhang LQ, Watson HG, et al. Hepatitis C quantification and sequencing in blood products, haemophiliacs, and drug users. Lancet 1990 ; 336 : 1469-72.

6. Kaneko S, Murakami S, Unoura M, *et al*. Quantitation of hepatitis C virus RNA by competitive polymerase chain reaction. J Med Virol 1992 ; 37 : 278-82.
7. Compton J. Nucleic acid sequence-based amplification. Nature 1991 ; 350 : 91-2.
8. Kievits T, van Gemen B, van Strijp D, *et al*. NASBA isothermal enzymatic in vitro nucleic acid amplification optimized for the diagnosis of HIV-1 infection. J Virol Methods 1991 ; 35 : 273-86.
9. Boom R, Sol CJ, Salimans MM, *et al*. Rapid and simple method for purification of nucleic acids. J Clin Microbiol 1990 ; 28 : 495-503.
10. Bukh J, Purcell RH, Miller RH. Importance of primer selection for the detection of hepatitis C virus RNA with the polymerase chain reaction assay. Proc Natl Acad Sci USA 1992 ; 89 : 187-91.
11. Cristiano K, Di Bisceglie AM, Hoofnagle JH, *et al*. Hepatitis C viral RNA in serum of patients with chronic non-A, non-B hepatitis : detection by the polymerase chain reaction using multiple primer sets. Hepatology 1991 ; 14 : 51-5.
12. Choo QL, Richman KH, Han JH, *et al*. Genetic organization and diversity of the hepatitis C virus. Proc Natl Acad Sci USA 1991 ; 88 : 2451-5.
13. Kato N, Hijikata M, Ootsuyama Y, *et al*. A structural protein encoded by the 5' region of the hepatitis C virus genome efficiently detects viral infection. Jpn J Cancer Res 1990 ; 81 : 1092-4.
14. Takamizawa A, Mori C, Fuke I, *et al*. Structure and organization of the hepatitis C virus genome isolated from human carriers. J Virol 1991 ; 65 : 1105-13.
15. Okamoto H, Okada S, Sugiyama Y, *et al*. Nucleotide sequence of the genomic RNA of hepatitis C virus isolated from a human carrier : comparison with reported isolates for conserved and divergent regions. J Gen Virol 1991 ; 72 : 2697-704.
16. Takeuchi K, Boonmar S, Kubo Y, *et al*. Hepatitis C viral cDNA clones isolated from a healthy carrier donor implicated in post-transfusion non-A, non-B hepatitis. Gene 1990 ; 91 : 287-91.
17. Chen PJ, Lin MH, Tu SJ, *et al*. Isolation of a complementary DNA fragment of hepatitis C virus in Taiwan revealed significant sequence variations compared with other isolates. Hepatology 1991 ; 14 : 73-8.
18. Inchauspe G, Zebedee S, Lee DH, *et al*. Genomic structure of the human prototype strain H of hepatitis C virus : comparison with American and Japanese isolates. Proc Natl Acad Sci USA 1991 ; 88 : 10292-6.
19. Chen PJ, Lin MH, Tai KF, *et al*. The Taiwanese hepatitis C virus genome : sequence determination and mapping the 5' termini of viral genomic and antigenomic RNA. Virology 1992 ; 188 : 102-13.
20. Okamoto H, Kurai K, Okada S, *et al*. Full-length sequence of a hepatitis C virus genome having poor homology to reported isolates : comparative study of four distinct genotypes. Virology 1992 ; 188 : 331-41.
21. Takeuchi K, Kubo Y, Boonmar S, *et al*. The putative nucleocapsid and envelope protein genes of hepatitis C virus determined by comparison of the nucleotide sequences of two isolates derived from an experimentally infected chimpanzee and healthy human carriers. J Gen Virol 1990 ; 71 : 3027-33.
22. Han JH, Shyamala V, Richman KH, *et al*. Characterization of the terminal regions of hepatitis C viral RNA : identification of conserved sequences in the 5' untranslated region and poly(A) tails at the 3' end. Proc Natl Acad Sci USA 1991 ; 88 : 1711-5.
23. Cha TA, Beall E, Irvine B, *et al*. At least five related, but distinct, hepatitis C viral genotypes exist. Proc Natl Acad Sci USA 1992 ; 89 : 7144-8.
24. Castillo I, Bartolome J, Quiroga JA, *et al*. Comparison of several PCR procedures for detection of serum HCV-RNA using different regions of the HCV genome. J Virol Methods 1992 ; 38 : 71-9.
25. Okamoto H, Okada S, Sugiyama Y, *et al*. Detection of hepatitis C virus RNA by a two-stage polymerase chain reaction with two pairs of primers deduced from the 5'-noncoding region. Jpn J Exp Med 1990 ; 60 : 215-22.
26. Garson JA, Ring C, Tuke P, *et al*. Enhanced detection by PCR of hepatitis C virus RNA. Lancet 1990 ; 336 : 878-9.

27. Bukh J, Purcell RH, Miller RH. Sequence analysis of the 5' noncoding region of hepatitis C virus. Proc Natl Acad Sci U S A 1992 ; 89 : 4942-6.
28. Stuyver L, Rossau R, Wyseur A, et al. Typing of hepatitis C virus isolates and characterization of new subtypes using a line probe assay. J Gen Virol 1993 ; 74 : 1093-102.
29. Simmonds P, McOmish F, Yap PL, et al. Sequence variability in the 5' non-coding region of hepatitis C virus : identification of a new virus type and restrictions on sequence diversity. J Gen Virol 1993 ; 74 : 661-8.
30. Owczarek CM, Enriquez-Harris P, Proudfoot NJ. The primary transcription of the human 2 globin gene defined by quantitative RT/PCR. Nuc Acids Res 1992 ; 20 : 851-8.
31. Holodniy M, Katzenstein DA, Sengupta S, et al. Detection and quantification of human immunodeficiency virus RNA in patient serum by use of the polymerase chain reaction. J Infect Dis 1991 ; 163 : 862-6.
32. Eron JJ, Gorzyca P, Kaplan JC, et al. Susceptibility testing by polymerase chain reaction DNA quantitation : A method to measure drug resistance of human immunodeficiency virus type 1 isolates. Proc Natl Acad Sci, USA 1992 ; 89 : 3241-5.
33. Brillanti S, Garson JA, Tuke PW, et al. Effect of alpha-interferon therapy on hepatitis C viraemia in community-acquired chronic non-A, non-B hepatitis : a quantitative polymerase chain reaction study. J Med Virol 1991 ; 34 : 136-41.
34. Garson JA, Brillanti S, Ring C, et al. Hepatitis C viraemia rebound after « successful » interferon therapy in patients with chronic non-A, non-B hepatitis. J Med Virol 1992 ; 37 : 210-4.
35. Hagiwara H, Hayashi N, Mita E, et al. Quantitative analysis of hepatitis C virus RNA in serum during interferon alfa therapy. Gastroenterology 1993 ; 104 : 877-83.
36. Nedelman J, Heagerty P, Lawrence C. Quantitative PCR : procedures and precisions. Bull Math Biology 1992 ; 54 : 477-502.
37. Nedelman J, Heagerty P, Lawrence C. Quantitative PCR with internal controls. Comput Appl Biosci 1992 ; 8 : 65-70.
38. Kenten JH, Gudibande S, Link J, et al. Improved electrochemiluminescent label for DNA probe assays : rapid quantitative assays of HIV-1 polymerase chain reaction products. Clin Chem 1992 ; 38 : 873-9.
39. Van Gemen B, Kievits T, Schukkink R, et al. Quantification of HIV-1 RNA in plasma using NASBA during HIV-1 primary infection. J Virol Methods 1993 ; 43 : 177-87.
40. Jurriaans S, Dekker JT, Ronde de A. HIV-1 viral DNA load in peripheral blood mononuclear cells from seroconverters and long-term infected individuals. AIDS 1992 ; 6 : 635-41.

8

Detection of HCV RNA in serum using a single-tube, single enzyme PCR in combination with a colorimetric microwell assay

L. WOLFE[1], S. TAMATSUKURI[2], C. SAYADA[3], J.-C. RYFF with the Viral Hepatitis Study Group[4]

[1] *Roche Molecular Systems, Branchburg, NJ.*
[2] *Nippon Roche, Tokyo, Japan.*
[3] *Roche Diagnostics, Paris, France.*
[4] *Department of International Clinical Research, Hoffmann-La Roche, Basel, Switzerland.*

Introduction

Hepatitis C virus is considered to be the principle etiologic agent responsible for 90-95 % of post-transfusion non-A, non-B hepatitis cases [1, 2]. HCV is single-stranded, positive sense RNA virus with a genome of approximately 10,000 nucleotides coding for 3,000 amino acids. As a blood-born virus, it may be transmitted by blood and blood products. Prevalence of HCV infection is high in patients receiving organ transplants, blood transfusions, or commercial clotting factors, in patients with percutaneous exposure through intravenous drug abuse, and in patients undergoing renal dialysis. The global prevalence of HCV infection, as determined by immunoserology, ranges from 0.6 % in Canada to 1.5 % in Japan [1].

The presence of anti-HCV antibodies in patients infected with HCV has led to the development of immunological assays currently approved for blood donor screening. Implementation of these assays already has reduced the incidence of post-transfusion hepatitis in the United States. Additional supplemental testing often is performed using the

RIBA (recombinant immunoblot assay) to further evaluate those samples that are repeatedly reactive samples. Recent evaluations have shown that interpretation of these immunological tests often is difficult since 25-90 % (depending on the risk group under evaluation) of samples repeatedly reactive in the screening assay are negative upon supplemental evaluation with the RIBA assay [2, 3].

Immunoserological testing is a measure of prior exposure HCV infection, but can not be considered a marker for current infection. At the present time, an immunological assay for direct detection of HCV antigen is unavailable. Furthermore, in cases of acute HCV resulting from accidental needlestick exposure, many patients fail to produce antibody to HCV [4] making diagnosis of HCV infection impossible using immunoserological techniques. On the other hand, detection of HCV viremia by PCR offers a marker of current infection. Using PCR, it has been possible to detect HCV viremia prior to immunological sero-conversion [5, 6], and to detect fluctuation of viremia in antibody-positive chronic HCV patients undergoing therapy with interferon [7]. Since PCR is able to amplify HCV RNA directly, independently of the patient's immunological status, a PCR-based assay also is valuable in detecting HCV RNA in immunocompromised patients.

Most previous approaches to PCR-based detection of HCV have utilized lengthy sample preparation procedures, a cumbersome two-step, two-enzyme combination for reverse transcription and nested PCR, and detection by agarose gels. We describe a simplified assay for the detection of HCV in human serum or plasma.

Methods

Sample preparation

Serum or plasma (ACD anti-coagulant) were collected from each patient within 30 minutes of blood draw and held at $-70\ °C$ until use. Analysis of each sample was performed using Amplicor™ HCV reagents. HCV RNA was isolated from serum using a modification of previously published procedures based on GuSCN and ethanol precipitation in the presence of poly rA carrier RNA, and amplified in an RNA PCR reaction equivalent to 5 μl serum/PCR.

Amplification conditions

For the amplification reaction, Amplicor™ HCV provides a Master Mix that contains the rTth DNA polymerase enzyme, a single primer pair, buffer salts, dATP, dCTP, dGTP, and dUTP. The latter, dUTP, is incorporated into each amplification product to serve as a a substrate for the AmpErase™ enzyme, Uracil N-glycosylase [12] to prevent carrier-over contamination of previously amplified material. A single primer pair, including a biotinylated downstream primer (KY 80 5'-GCAGAAAGCGTCTAGCCATGGCGT, and KY78 5'-Biotinyl-CTCGCAAGCACCCTATCAGGCAGT) defines an amplicon located in the 5'-untranslated region of HCV for the amplification of a highly conserved sequence. We have optimized reaction conditions for the use of the rTth DNA polymerase which, in the presence of manganese performs both reverse transcription and DNA polymerase functions, obviating the requirement for two enzymes or for two separate reactions. With the thermally stable rTth enzyme, reverse transcription may be performed at elevated temperatures as high as 60-70 °C. Amplification is carried out in the Perkin-Elmer thermal-cycler 9600 with a program that allows for a 2 minute incubation at 50 degrees (for optimal AmpErase activity to form single-stranded nicks in previously amplified product containing dUTP), followed by a 30 minute incubation at 60 degrees (for the reverse-transcriptase step, and 40 cycles of PCR.

Detection of amplification products

Detection of the PCR product is accomplished with an added level of specificity through the use of a solid phase probe specific for HCV that is coated onto microwell plates. The PCR product (labeled through the 5'-biotinylated downstream primer) is hybridized to the microwell and detected using an avidin-horse radish peroxidase system using conventional microtiter plate washer and microtiter plate reader (450 nm). Using these methods, the time to result is approximately 6 hours for a batch-size of 25 samples. Alternatively, if samples are already extracted, up to 96 samples (including Positive and Negative controls) may be analyzed in the same period of time (Figure 1).

Study Design for Japanese Evaluation

A clinical evaluation of Amplicor™ HCV was performed on 294 serum samples collected at Tokyo University, Chiba University, and Kurume University in Japan. Each site was asked to collect

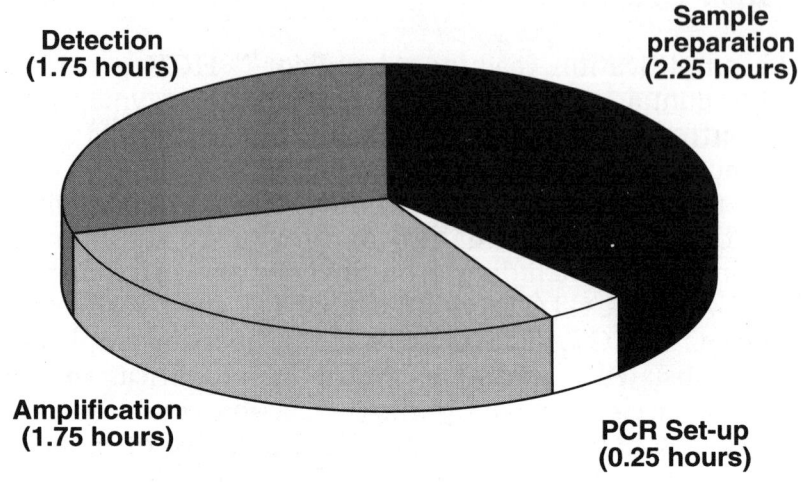

Figure 1. Time to result for Amplicor™ HCV assay. A batch size of 25 samples can be extracted, amplified, and detected in approximately 6 hours. Alternatively, up to 96 samples, already extracted, can be analyzed in the same amount of time.

approximately 100 sera, of which approximately 70 % were to be HCV antibody positive, and approximately 30 % were to have liver disease of other origin (Hepatitis A or B, alcoholic cirrhosis, hepatocellular carcinoma, or other organ disease. From each identified patient, blood was drawn into each of two Serum Separator Tubes (B-D). Both tubes were allowed to clot for 30 minutes after the blood draw, centrifuged, and frozen at − 80 degrees Centigrade immediately. For each sample, both SST tubes were delivered frozen to Nippon Roche, Kamakura Laboratory, where one of the tubes was thawed and immediately analyzed using Amplicor HCV. The duplicate tube was delivered frozen, never thawed, to a commercial laboratory for PCR evaluation using a PCR protocol based on MuLV RT/Taq polymerase PCR using 5'UTR nested-primers and agarose gel detection.

Results

The analytical sensitivity of this assay is shown in Figure 2 as a function of PCR cycle number (2-a) and dilution of amplicon applied to the microwell detection assay (2-b). It can be seen that this assay readily detects 10 input copies of an HCV RNA transcript after 40 amplification cycles. However, under these conditions, the optical

HCV Amplicon formation as a function of cycle number
(Microwell Analysis Of Undiluted Amplicon)

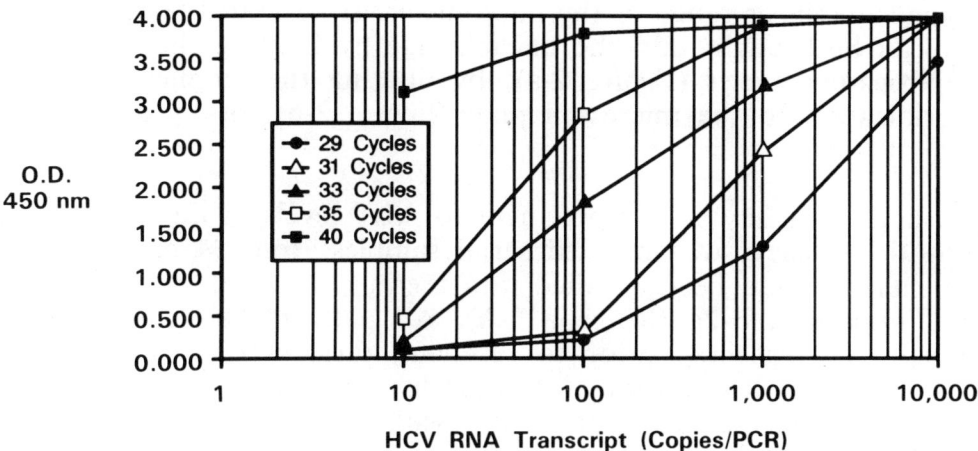

Figures 2-a and 2-b. Analytical Sensitivity of the Amplicor™ assay. An HCV RNA transcript spanning the 5' UTR and part of the core gene was characterized for input copy number using Poisson analysis. Input HCV RNA transcript ranging from 10-10,000 copies were amplified as described using 29-40 PCR cycles and hybridized to microwell plates using undiluted amplicon (2-a). The effect of diluting the amplicon produced from 35 cycles of PCR, prior to hybridization to the microwell plate, can be seen in (2-b).

Dilution of HCV Amplicon
35 Cycles Of PCR

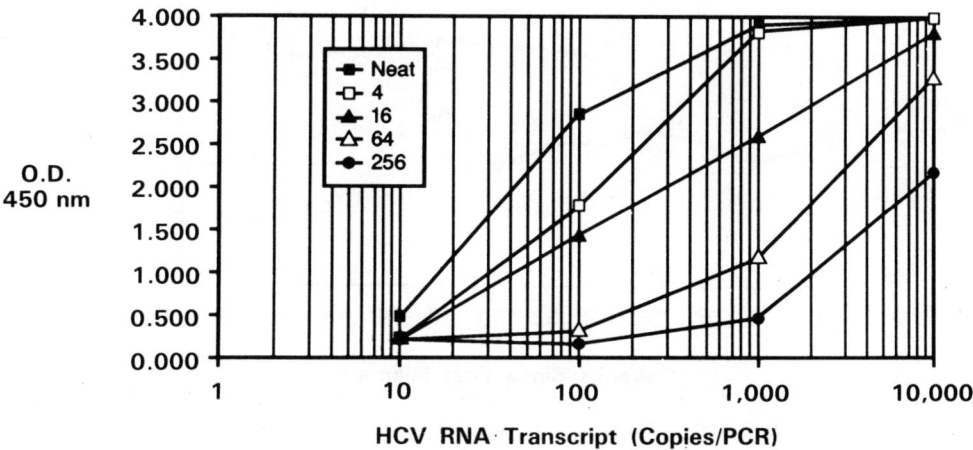

density obtained from amplification of as few as 10 copies is well beyond the linear range of the photometer. If desired, the optical density can be brought into the linear range by limiting the number of amplification cycles (Figure 2-a), by diluting the amplicon prior to hybridization to the microwell plate (Figure 2-b), or by a combination of both.

Using this assay as a supplement to ALT levels in monitoring therapeutic efficacy, we analyzed serial samples from 44 chronic HCV patients who had been enrolled in a therapy protocol using recombinant interferon α-2a (Roferon™-A). All patients had chronic HCV infection at baseline, prior to receiving thrice-weekly injections of Roferon-A for a duration of 12 months. Patients were followed for 18 months after beginning of therapy with measurement of ALT levels and PCR determination of viremia at approximately two-month intervals. In this selected group of 44 patients, there were 14 responders (either normal ALT levels, or absence of HCV RNA in serum for at least 2 months at the completion of the study), and 30 non-responders (including 1 placebo). Figure 3 shows the placebo case with persistant elevation of ALT levels throughout the study, and the continuing pre-

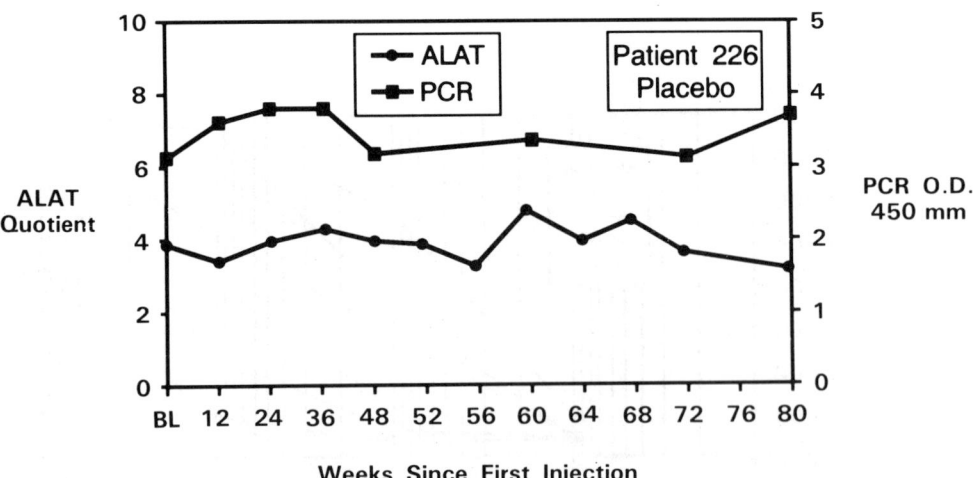

Figure 3. Response to interferon therapy-a placebo profile.

sence of HCV viremia, as determined by PCR. On the other hand, 7 of the 14 responders to therapy showed the following pattern — within 3 months of therapy, ALT levels normalized, and HCV RNA became undetectable by PCR (not shown). Five of the responders required periods longer than 3 months for both ALT and HCV levels to decline (Figure 4), and 2 of the 14 responded by ALT criteria alone — ALT levels had normalized at the completion of the study, although the patient was still viremic, as determined by PCR (Figure 5).

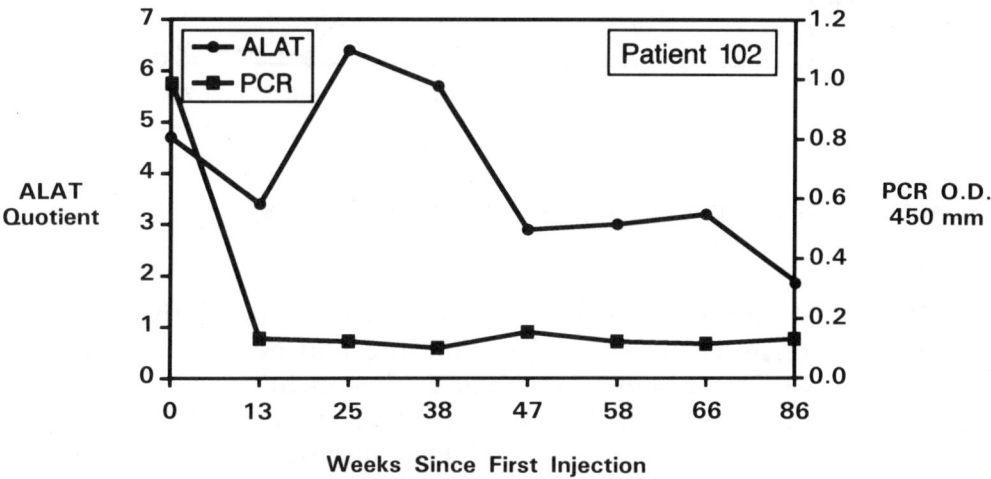

Figure 4. Elevated ALT levels in the absence of viremia.

Of the 30 non-responders, 4 patients responded initially by both ALT and PCR criteria, remained apparently normal for greater than 24 weeks, and ultimately relapsed by both ALT and PCR criteria when therapy was discontinued at the end of the study (Figure 6). The rest of the non-responders exhibited fluctuating ALT levels generally correlating with fluctuations in levels of HCV RNA.

This assay also was evaluated for its utility as a differential diagnostic tool in an infectious disease environment. PCR analysis was performed using Amplicor™ HCV in comparison to a nested PCR method used commercially in Japan on 294 samples whose serological status was known. This patient population for this evaluation inclu-

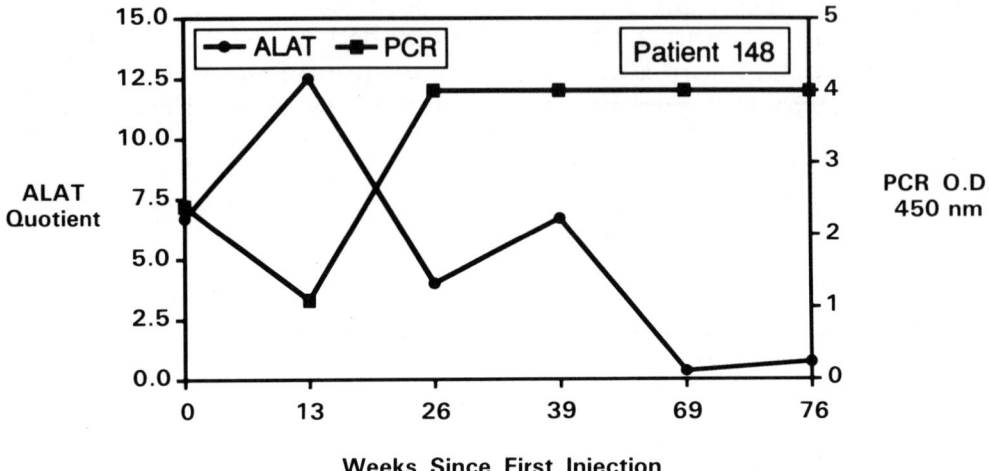

Figure 5. Viremia in the absence of elevated ALT levels.

ded 211 HCV sero-positive patients. Of these sero-positive patients, 89 had been on interferon therapy, and 122 had never been on interferon therapy. This patient population also included 83 HCV sero-negative patients — 3 with documented HAV infection, 26 with documented HBV infection, 14 with fatty liver disease, 39 with other liver disease, and 1 normal patient.

The specificity of the assay, compared to that of nested PCR is shown in Figure 7. All 83 HCV sero-negative patients were negative using the Amplicor™ HCV assay. On the other hand, the nested PCR method gave 5 positive results in this population. These 5 results are interpreted as false-positive results attributed to the prevalence of carry-over contamination with the nested-PCR method.

The clinical sensitivity of Amplicor™ HCV is shown in Figure 8. Again, all of the sero-negative patients were PCR negative. Of 11 sero-positive patients, 176 were positive using Amplicor™ HCV. Thirty-five patients were sero-positive, but PCR negative. However, 30 of these patients had been on interferon therapy, 2 patients had hepatocellular carcinoma, and 1 patient had alcoholic cirrhosis.

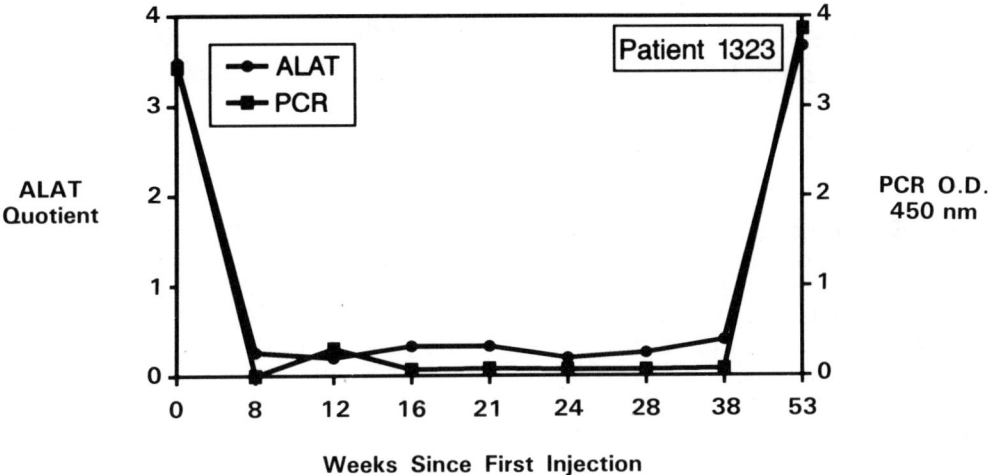

Figure 6. Relapse as determined by both ALT and PCR criteria. Serial samples from patients undergoing 12 months of therapy with recombinant interferon α-2a (Roferon™ were evaluated for ALT levels, and for viremia, as determined by PCR. Varied response patterns included placebo and non-responder (Figure 3), elevated ALT levels in the absence of viremia (Figure 4), viremia in the absence of elevated ALT levels (Figure 5), and relapse at the end of therapy (Figure 6).

		HAV	HBV	Fatty Liver Disease	Other Liver Disease	Normal
Amplicor HCV	+	0	0	0	0	0
	−	3	26	14	39	1
RT-nested PCR	+	0	3	1	1	0
	−	3	23	13	38	1

Figure 7. Specificity of Amplicor HCV compared to nested PCR. Patients with liver disease of various origins were handled as previously described for the Japanese evaluation. Shown in Figure 7 are 83 patients with liver disease, all of whom were sero-negative for HCV — 3 with documented HAV infection, 26 with documented HBV infection, 14 with fatty liver disease, 39 with other liver disease, and 1 normal patient. All 83 patients were negative by Amplicor™ HCV.

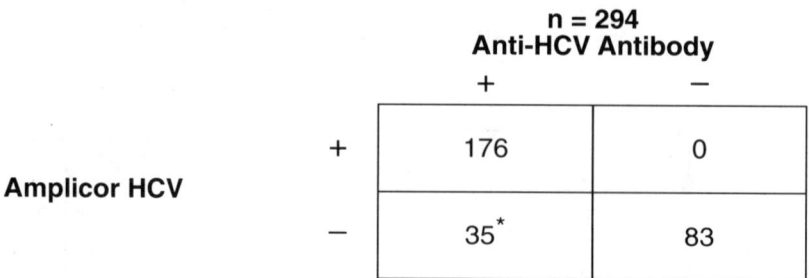

Figure 8. Clinical Sensitivity of Amplicor™ HCV compared to immunoserology. Patients with liver disease of various origins were handled as previously described for the Japanese evaluation. Shown is a comparison of immunoserology and PCR results for 294 patients. All 83 sero-negative patients were PCR negative, as also shown in Figure 6. Of 211 sero-positive patients, 176 were positive using Amplicor™ HCV. Thirty-five patients were sero-positive, but PCR negative — including 30 who had been on interferon therapy, 2 with hepatocellular carcinoma, and 1 with alcoholic cirrhosis.

The concordance of nested PCR and Amplicor™ HCV was generally quite good — 168 samples were positive in both PCR assays. Eight samples which were positive by Amplicor™ HCV, but negative by nested PCR, were all from HCV sero-positive patients with documented chronic HCV infection, suggesting a higher clinical sensitivity for Amplicor™ HCV. Five of nine samples which were Amplicor™ HCV negative, but positive by nested PCR, were from sero-negative individuals with no history of HCV infection and, as suggested above, may be false positive results due to the technical problems associated with the nested PCR approach. The remaining 4 samples which were Amplicor™ HCV negative, but positive by nested PCR, were from chronic HCV patients undergoing interferon therapy.

Discussion

This HCV PCR assay is a single-tube, single polymerase, single primer pair approach to the detection of HCV RNA in serum with a sensitivity of 10-100 input copies/PCR. Although qualitative in nature, this assay has been used as an aid to monitor efficacy of interferon therapy. Although PCR detection of HCV RNA in the serum generally correlates well with ALT level (in 7 interferon reponders, and in 21 non-responders), neither PCR nor ALT level alone givies a complete profile of a patient's status. A fall in ALT levels often lagged behind a decline in viremia. Furthermore, we have observed both elevated ALT levels in the absence of HCV RNA, and HCV viremia in the presence of normal ALT levels. More extensive evaluations will be needed to determine the prognostic value of viremia as determined by PCR.

Similarly, the evaluation of Amplicor™ HCV as a differential diagnostic tool has shown this to be an assay of high positive predictive value. The specificity of the assay for use with liver disease patients was shown to be excellent. Furthermore, the clinical sensitivity of this assay appears to be higher than for some nested PCR approaches currently in use. Figures 2a and 2b emphasize the assay parameters that can be manipulated into a more quantitative format. A more quantitative approach could allow more flexibility in tailoring more aggressive anti-viral approaches to those patients with higher viral titers at baseline. Currently, such a semi-quantitative approach, incorporating an internal amplification control, is under evalution.

References

1. Alter H. Descartes before the horse : I clone, therefore I am : the hepatitis C virus in current perspective. Ann Intern Med 1991 ; 115 : 644-9.
2. McHutchison J, Person J, Govindarajan S, *et al*. Improved detection of hepatitis C virus antibodies in high-risk populations. Hepatology 1992 ; 15 : 19-25.
3. Chaudray RK, Andonov A, Mac Lean C. Detection of hepatitis C virus infection with recombinant immunoblot assay, synthetic immunoblot assay, and polymerase chain reaction. J Clin Lab Anal 1993 ; 7 : 164-7.
4. Mitsui T, Iwano K, Masuko K, *et al*. Hepatitis C virus infection in medical personnel after needlestick accident. Hepatology 1992 ; 16 : 1109-14.
5. Puoti M, Zonaro A, Ravagii, *et al*. Hepatitis C virus RNA and antibody response in the clinical course of acute hepatitis C virus infection. Hepatology 1992 ; 16 : 877-81.
6. Young K, Resnick R, Myers T. Detection of hepatitis C virus RNA by a combined reverse transcriptase-polymerase chain reaction assay. J Clin Microbiol 1993 ; 31 : 882-6.
7. Shindo M, Bisceglie A, Cheung L, *et al*. Decrease in serum hepatitis C viral RNA during alpha-interferon therapy for chronic hepatitis C. Ann Intern Med 1991 ; 115 : 700-4.
8. Stuyver L, Rossau R, Wyseur A, *et al*. Typing of hepatitis C virus isolates and characterization of new sub-types using a line probe assay. J Gen Virol 1993 ; 74 : 1093-102.
9. Machida A, Ohnuma H, Tsuda F, *et al*. Two distinct subtypes of hepatitis C virus defined by antibodies directed to the putative core protein. Hepatology 1992 ; 16 : 886-91.
10. Bukh J, Purcell, Miller R. Importance of primer selection for the detection of hepatitis C virus RNA with the polymerase chain reaction. Proc Natl Acad Sci USA 1992 ; 89 : 187-91.

11. Okamoto H, Okada S, Sugiyama Y, *et al*. The 5'-terminal sequence of the hepatitis C virus genome. Japan. J Exp Med 1990 ; 60 : 167-77.
12. Longo MC, MS Beringer, Hartley JL. Use of uracil DNA glycosylase to control carry-over contamination in polymerase chain reactions. Gene 93, 1990 ; 125-8.

9

Quantitation of serum hepatitis C virus RNA by branched DNA amplification and distribution of HCV genotypes in anti-HCV positive blood donors

P. MARCELLIN, M. MARTINOT-PEIGNOUX, J. GOURNAY, J.-P. BENHAMOU, S. ERLINGER

Service d'Hépatologie et INSERM U24, Hôpital Beaujon, Clichy, France.

It is generally admitted that the presence of hepatitis C virus (HCV) replication is usually correlated to increased serum alanine aminotransferase (ALT) levels [1]. Until recently, only polymerase chain reaction (PCR) could provide evidence for active HCV replication [2]. The recent study by Zaaijer et al. [3] indicates the poor reliability of HCV-PCR. Indeed only 16 % of the laboratories participating in that study performed HCV-PCR faultlessly. Furthermore, the level of HCV replication cannot be quantitated by PCR. A new approach, called branched DNA (bDNA) signal amplification, has recently been developed and can be used to quantitate serum HCV RNA [4]. The recent study by Lau et al. showed that the level of HCV RNA may have some clinical relevance in patients with chronic hepatitis C [5]. However, these patients are only a subgroup of the overall population with chronic HCV infection. Blood donors with antibodies to HCV antigens (anti-HCV) are probably more representative of the spectrum of subjects infected with HCV. Furthermore, partial and entire sequences of various HCV isolates have been determined : there were divergent sequences among distinct isolates [6-11]. The 5' non coding (5'NC) region is the most conserved among different isolates and the less conserved are the genome domaines E1 and E2/NS1 which encode proteins of the virion envelope [12, 13]. Significant genetic heterogeneity has been reported among isolates from different geographic areas and among isolates from the same individual [14]. From the sequence data, according to the sequences homology, the classification of the strains into four distinct types I, II, III and IV has been proposed by Okamoto [9]. Sequence diversity within the same genotype of HCV is less than 10 %. Most isolates described in Europe and USA belong to genotype I and genotype II, while most of those described in Japan belong to genotype II, genotype III and genotype IV, which suggests that the 4 genotypes of HCV segregate geographically.

The objective of this study was to assess HCV replication and HCV genotypes in blood donors who were anti-HCV positive and PCR positive for HCV RNA. HCV replication was assessed by quantitation of serum HCV RNA with bDNA signal amplification and HCV genotypes were determined by restriction length fragment polymorphism. In addition, we evaluated the relation between serum HCV RNA level, HCV genotype, epidemiological characteristics and serum ALT levels.

Patients and methods

Fifty four anti-HCV positive blood donors consecutively seen at the outpatient clinics of the department of Hepatology (Hôpital Beaujon) were studied. These blood donors were systematically referred from three Blood Centers in the Hôpital Beaujon area located in the Northern suburbs of Paris. Anti-HCV were screened with third generation ELISA (ELISA3) (Ortho Diagnostic Systems, Roissy, France) and confirmed with third generation RIBA (RIBA3) (Ortho Diagnostic Systems, Roissy, France). There were 25 females and 29 males, mean age 37 years (range 22 to 64). Risk factors were found in 42 subjects (blood transfusion in 16, intravenous drug addiction in 23, professionnal exposure in 3). Twenty one had normal serum ALT levels and 33 had serum ALT levels above the upper limit of the normal range (40 IU/L) on the day of serum collection.

HCV RNA detection was performed by PCR with primers located in the 5' non-coding region of the HCV genome [15]. HCV RNA quantitation was performed with the quantitative bDNA signal amplification assay (Quantiplex Chiron Diagnostics, Lyon, France) on serum aliquoted and frozen at -20 °C within 2 hours after collection. This assay is based on specific hybridization of synthetic oligonucleotides located in the 5' untranslated region of the HCV genome which allows the HCV RNA to be captured onto the surface of a well. Synthetic branched DNA molecules (dDNA) and multiple copies of an alkaline phosphatase-linked probe are hybridized to the immobilized complex. Detection is achieved by incubation with a chemiluminescent substrate (Dioxetane) and measurement of the light emission, the signal being proportional to the amount of the target RNA captured. The limit of detection (cut-off) of the assay is 3.5×10^5 copies HCV genome equivalent per ml (Eq/ml). The samples are run in duplicate and if the coefficient of variation (CV) is greater than 20 % the assay must be repeated. This standardized method allows to test 42 patients in one overnight hybridization and 3 hours revelation.

HCV genotyping was performed in the NS5 region of the HCV genome with restriction length fragment polymorphism [16] (RLFP) in the 36 blood donors found PCR positive with primers located in this region of the HCV genome. A computer analysis of available sequences date [6, 8] was done to construct restriction maps for the amplified NS5 fragment of HCV genome and to choose restriction endonucleases. Restriction endonuclease *Alu*I and *Sau*96I were the most discriminants to distinguish the HCV genotypes. The *Alu*I or *Sau*96I restriction maps for the amplified NS5 fragment were determined with the following four isolates [17] : HCV-PT (genotype I), HCV K1 (genotype II), HCV K2a (genotype III) and HCV K2b (genotype IV).

StatView SE + Graphic program (Abacus Concepts, Berkeley, USA) with correlation was used as well as Mann-Whitney's and Krushal-Wallis non-parametric tests as appropriate. To ensure that none of the associations were dependent on the computation level, the analysis was performed twice with the lower cut-off values set at zero and 1×10^5 Eq/ml level.

Results

All the 54 blood donors had by definition serum HCV RNA detectable with PCR. Serum HCV RNA was detected with bDNA signal amplification in 42 of the 54 blood donors (77 %) at levels ranging from cut-off to 259×10^5 Eq/ml. One donor was indeterminate and 11 (3 with normal serum ALT and 8 with increased serum ALT levels) were below the cut-off. None had a CV greater than 20 %.

Genotype I, II and III were found in 19, 14 and 3 blood donors respectively. No patient had genotype IV. The median values were 39.9×10^5 Eq/ml (range: cut-off to 87.6×10^5 Eq/ml) and 28.8×10^5 Eq/ml (range: cut-off to 180×10^5 Eq/ml) in subjects with genotypes I and II, respectively (difference not significant) (Table I).

Table I. Serum HCV RNA levels according to HCV genotype in the 36 blood donors.

Genotype	I	II	III
Number of patients	19	14	3
Serum HCV RNA ($\times 10^5$ Eq/ml)			
Median	39.5	28.8	< 3.5
Range	cut-off-87.6	cut-off-180	cut-off-14.7

The median values were 14.7×10^5 Eq/ml (range: cut-off to 259×10^5 Eq/ml) and 28.6×10^5 Eq/ml (range: cut-off to 180×10^5 Eq/ml) in the 21 blood donors with normal and the 33 blood donors with increased serum ALT levels, respectively (no significant difference). There was no significant correlation between serum ALT levels and serum HCV RNA levels ($r = 0.19$) (Figure 1).

There was no relationship between the source of infection and the levels of HCV RNA. The median values were: 17×10^5 Eq/ml (range: cut-off to 180×10^5 Eq/ml), 28.4×10^5 Eq/ml (range: cut-off to 259×10^5 Eq/ml) and 26.6×10^5 Eq/ml (range: cut-off to 173×10^5 Eq/ml) in subjects with community acquired, blood transfusion and drug addiction related infection, respectively (Table II). No correlation was found between age or sex ratios and the level of HCV RNA.

Table II. Serum HCV RNA levels according to source of infection in 51 blood donors.

	Community acquired	Blood transfusion	Drug addiction
Number of patients	12	16	23
Serum HCV RNA ($\times 10^5$ Eq/ml)			
Median	17	28.4	26.6
Range	cut-off-180	cut-off-255	cut-off-173

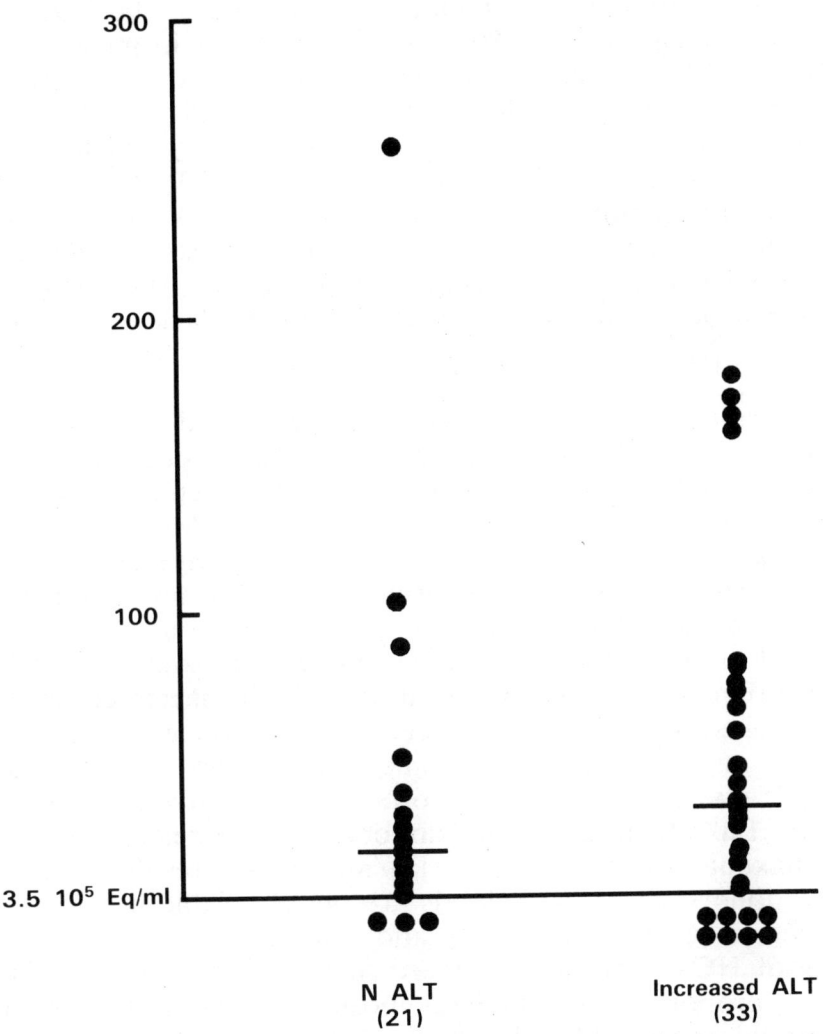

Figure 1. Serum HCV RNA quantitation according to ALT level.

Discussion

The measurements of serum HCV RNA levels in this study are probably a good reflection of the amount of circulating serum HCV RNA since these results correspond to the 72 % positivity rate found by Lau et al. [5] in a population of 48 patients with chronic hepatitis C and the 82 % positivity rate found by Bresters et al. [17] in a mixed population of 50 haemophiliacs or blood donors. Thus, the bDNA signal amplification identifies true HCV viremic subjects in most but not all PCR positive blood donors probably because of a titer of serum HCV RNA which is below the limit of detection (3.5×10^5 Eq/ml) of this assay. Branched DNA signal amplification assay which has a good reliability could be used as a screening assay and PCR because of its high sensitivity should be performed in anti-HCV positive subjects found negative with bDNA signal amplification assay. The combination of these two techniques might be hepfull in, resolving the problems which occur with contamination and the lack of reliability [3] of PCR.

These results show that in a population of blood donors with HCV RNA detectable with PCR, the level of HCV replication, measured with a quantitative method, is not correlated to, epidemiological characteristics such as sex, age or source of infection. Most of these results support those of Lau et al. [5]. except for the age of the subjects. It is particularly interesting that serum HCV RNA levels were not correlated to serum ALT levels. Indeed, the proportion of the blood donors with normal serum ALT levels and detectable serum HCV RNA was not different from that of blood donors with increased serum ALT levels. Furthermore, the level of HCV replication was not correlated to the level of serum ALT, since some blood donors with normal serum ALT levels may have higher titers of serum HCV RNA (maximal value 259×10^5 Eq/ml) than blood donors with increased serum ALT levels (maximal value 180×10^5 Eq/ml). These results indicate that in blood donors serum ALT levels are not a reliable predictive factor of the degree of HCV infectivity and cannot be used as a marker of the level of HCV replication. Indeed, it has been shown that a relatively large proportion of anti-HCV positive symptom-free individuals with normal serum ALT levels have histologic lesions of chronic hepatitis [18].

By analyzing the NS5 region of the viral genome using PCR and RFLP analysis, we found in this population the presence of the three distinct genotypes of HCV, HCV genotypes I, II and III, but we found no subject infected by HCV genotype IV. Genotypes I and II were predominant (53 % and 39 % respectively) and genotype III was minoritary (8 %). As in previous studies in Western countries, we found that genotype I (close to the US isolate) was predominant in France [10, 11]. We also found a high proportion of isolates from genotype II : the use of Japanese primers for genotyping could have favoured the amplification of genotypes closely related to Japanese strains. We found no correlation between HCV genotype and the amount of circulating HCV RNA which suggests that the level of HCV replication, is not clearly related to HCV genotype. However these measurements on a single serum may not reflect the fluctuations of circulating HCV RNA.

In conclusion, our results suggest that there is no correlation between serum HCV RNA levels and HCV genotypes at least with genotypes I or II more frequently found in western Europe. The level of HCV replication does not seem to be correlated to serum ALT levels.

Aknowledgements : we thank Dr JP Bonn (Chiron, France) and Dr P Aumont (Ortho Diagnostic Systems, Roissy, France) for providing the Quantiplex and the anti-HCV tests.

References

1. Van der Poel CL, Reesink HW, Schaaberg L, *et al*. Infectivity of blood seropositive for hepatitis C virus antibodies. Lancet 1990 ; 335 : 558-60.
2. Weiner AJ, Kuo G, Bradley DW, *et al*. Detection of hepatitis C viral sequence in non-A, non-B hepatitis. Lancet 1990 ; 335 : 317-9.
3. Zaaijer HL, Cuypers HTM, Reesink HW, *et al*. Reliability of polymerase chain reaction for detection of hepatitis C virus. Lancet 1993 ; 341 : 722-4.
4. Urdea MS, Horn T, Fulz TJ, *et al*. Branched DNA amplification multimers for the sensitive direct detection of human hepatitis viruses. Nucl Acids Res Symp Ser 1991 ; 24 : 197-200.
5. Lau JY, Davis GL, Kniffen J, *et al*. Significance of serum hepatitis C virus RNA levels in chronic hepatitis. Lancet 1993 ; 341 : 1501-4.
6. Choo QL, Richman KH, Han JH, *et al*. Genetic organization and diversity of the hepatitis C virus. Proc Natl Acad Sci USA 1991 ; 88 : 2451-5.
7. Kato N, Hijikata M, Ootsuyama Y, Nakagawa M, Ohkoshi S, Sugimura T, Shimotohno K. Molecular cloning of the human hepatitis C virus genome from Japanese patients with non-A, non-B hepatitis. Proc Natl Acad Sci USA 1990 ; 87 : 9524-8.
8. Enomoto N, Takada A, Nakao T, Date T. There are two major types of hepatitis C virus in Japan. Biochem Biophys Res Commun 1990 ; 170 : 1021-5.
9. Okamoto H, Kurai K, Okada S, *et al*. Full-lenght sequence of a hepatitis C virus genome having poor homology to reported isolates comparative study of four distinct genotypes. Virology 1992 ; 188 : 331-41.
10. Kremsdorf D, Porchon C, Kim JP, Reyes GR, Brechot C. Partial nucleotide sequence analysis of a French hepatitis C virus implication for HCV genetic variability in the E2/NS1 protein. J Gen Virol 1991 ; 72 : 2557-61.
11. Li JS, Tong SP, Vitvitski L, Lepot D, Trépo C. Two French genotypes of hepatitis C virus homology of the predominant genotype with the prototype Americain strain. Gene 1991 ; 105 : 167-72
12. Weiner AJ, Brauer MJ, Rosenblatt J, *et al*. Variable and hypervariable domains are found in the regions of HCV corresponding to the Flavivirus envelope and NS1 proteins and the pestivirus envelope glycoproteins. Virology 1991 ; 180 : 842-7.

13. Houghton M, Weiner A, Han J, Kuo G, Choo QL. Molecular biology of the hepatitis C viruse implication for diagnosis, development and control of viral disease. Hepatology 1991 ; 14 : 381-8.
14. Ogata N, Alter HJ, Miller RH, Purcell RH. Nucleotide sequence and mutation rate of the H strain of hepatitis C virus. Proc Natl Acad Sci USA 1991 ; 88 : 3392-6.
15. Martinot-Peignoux M, Marcellin P, Xu LZ, *et al.* Reactivity to c33c antigen as a marker of hepatitis C virus multiplication. J Infect Dis 1992 ; 165 : 595-6.
16. Nakao T, Enomoto N, Takada A, *et al.* Typing hepatitis C virus genome by restriction fragment length polymorphisme. J Gen Virol 1991 ; 72 : 2105-12.
17. Bresters D, Mauser-Bunschoten EP, Reesink HW, *et al.* Sexual transmission of hepatitis C virus. Lancet 1993 ; 342 : 210-1.
18. Alberti A, Morsica G, Chemello L, *et al.* Hepatitis C vireamia and liver disease in symptom-free individuals with anti-HCV. Lancet 1992 ; 340 : 697-8.

10

Viremia, a more interesting factor than HCV genotype in chronic hepatitis C for predictive response to alpha-interferon therapy

M.-A. THELU[1], V. BARLET[1], M. COHARD[1,2], J.-M. SEIGNEURIN[1], J.-P. ZARSKI[1,2]

[1] Laboratoire de Virologie Médicale Moléculaire.
[2] Service d'Hépato-gastro-entérologie I, CHU, Grenoble, France.

Hepatitis C virus (HCV) is recognized as a major causative agent of non-A, non-B hepatitis. Molecular characterization of HCV genome revealed an RNA molecule of positive polarity of about 9,400 nucleotides (nt), including a 340 nt 5' untranslated region (5'UR), a long ORF which encodes a polyprotein of 3,011 amino acids [1, 2] and a short 3' untranslated region of variable length [1, 3]. The genome organization indicates a close relationship to the Pestiviridae and Flaviviridae. Different isolates of HCV show substantial nucleotide sequence variability distributed throughout the viral genome [4]. This degree of sequence variability is sufficient to alter the antigenic and biological properties of members of this virus group significantly. On the basis of these variations in nucleotide sequences, HCV has been classified into several groups. A phylogenetic tree of HCV containing four branches (ie : type I = HCV — 1 and HCV — H ; type II = HCV-J, -BK, HC-J4 ; type III : HC-J6 ; type IV : HC-J8) was proposed by Okamoto et al. [5] corresponding respectively to type 1a, 1b, 2a, 2b according to a classification proposed by McOmish et al. [6] and Simmonds et al. [7]. Recently, Okamoto et al. identified a new type V or 3a genotype from sera from NZL-1, Th 85, US 114 and HEM 26 isolats [8]. Serotype specific immunodominant epitopes have recently been mapped to the NS4 region of HCV [9]. This region contains a nonstructural viral protein of unknown fonction. Peptides based on these sequences have been used to develop an enzyme-linked immunosorbent assay that can serologically differentiate infections with three major types of HCV (type 1, 2 and 3) prevalent in European countries. Interferon (IFN) has been widely used in the treatment of chronic hepatitis C [10, 11]. There is some evidence for variation in the course of infection associated with different HCV variants and in response to treatment with interferon [12-15]. Moreover, HCV RNA detected by reverse transcription polymerase chain reaction (RT-PCR) can provide direct evidence for active viremia [16] but is not quantitative. Several cases have shown no improvement of serum ALT concentration despite the presence of low level hepatitis C viremia before interferon therapy [17]. A new approach to detect nucleic acid directly in clinical samples at the physiological concentrations by means of a signal amplification (branched DNA = bDNA) has been developed [18].

In our study, to investigate the relationship between serum HCV RNA levels of chronic hepatitis C patients treated with alpha-IFN and different factors, we detected presence of HCV RNA in serum by RT-PCR in the 5' UR, quantitated serum HCV RNA titers by bDNA in the 5' UR and determined HCV subtypes by Okamoto and Inno-LiPA methods. Okamoto method for typing HCV was developed, depending on the amplification of a C gene sequence by PCR using a universal primer (sense) and a mixture of five type-specific primers (antisense). HCV types were determined by the size of the products specific to each of them. Inno-LiPA method was developed for typing HCV in the 5'UTR. PCR amplification using biotinylated primers and type-specific probe on a Line Probe Assay (LiPA). We studied 34 patients with anti-HCV positive antibodies, but only 31 were treated with alpha-IFN. 3 asymptomatic carriers, 5 patients whose ALT normalized during or after therapy and remained so for more than 2 years, 9 patients whose ALT levels remained more than 1,5 times the upper limit of normal range during IFN-α administration were regarded as non responders (NR = group 5), 17 patients whose ALT levels fell below 1,5 times the upper limit of normal range during therapy but did not remain normal before the end of the treatment (9 early relapsers (ER = group 3)) or at the end of the treatment (8 later relapsers (LR = group 4)) were considered as partial responders.

When we compared the Okamoto and LiPA methods, the agreement was 70.6 % with a better relationship between mono-infected patients (82.6 %) ; indeed Inno-LiPA method did not detected multi-infections. After cloning and sequencing in the Core region serum sample of two patients with discordances, the Okamoto method was confirmed.

During the course of treatment, the genotype of patients was not modified. Indeed no selected genotype appeared.

Meanwhile, epidemiological characteristics showed a statistical correlation between type II and patients rather old, of female sex, and without drug addiction. Patients with type V were all drug abusers.

For multi-infected patients, viremia seemed lower and disease duration longer than those of mono-infected. Viremia seemed to be the best factor of predictive response to treatment with interferon.

In conclusion, our study suggests that there was no great difference between Okamoto and Inno-LiPA methods ; Okamoto method was time consuming but LiPA did not detect multi-infections. Better method will be well determined when we studied also serotyping. In our study, with low number of patients, no major genotype was associated with response to IFN α therapy. In chronic hepatitis C, viremia seemed to be a better factor than genotype for good response to IFN α therapy.

References

1. Kato N, Hijikata M, Ootsuyama Y, Nakagawa M, Ohkoshi S, Sugimura T, Shimotohno K. Molecular cloning of the human hepatitis C virus genome from japanese patients with non-A, non-B hepatitis. Proc Natl Acad Sci USA 1990 ; 87 : 9524-28.
2. Choo QL, Richman KH, Han JH, et al. Genetic organization and diversity of the hepatitis C virus. Proc Natl Acad Sci USA 1991 ; 88 : 2451-5.
3. Han JH, Shyamala V, Richman H, et al. Characterization of the terminal regions of hepatitis C viral RNA : identification of conserved sequences in the 5' untranslated region and poly (A) tails at the 3' end. Proc Natl Acad Sci USA 1991 ; 88 : 1711-5.
4. Okamoto H, Okada S, Sugiyama Y, et al. Nucleotide sequence of the genomic RNA of hepatitis C virus isolated from a human carrier : comparison with reported isolates for conserved and divergent regions. J Gen Virol 1991 ; 72 : 2697-704.
5. Okamoto H, Sugiyama Y, Okada S, et al. Typing hepatitis C virus by polymerase chain reaction with type-specific primers : application to clinical surveys and tracing infectious sources. J Gen Virol 1992 ; 73 : 673-9.

6. McOmish F, Chan SW, Dow BC, et al. Detection of three types of hepatitis C virus in blood donors : investigation of type-specific differences in serologic reactivity and rate of alanine aminotransferase abnormalities. Transfusion 1993 ; 33 : 7-13.
7. Simmonds P, McOmish F, Yap PL, et al. Sequence variability in the 5' non-coding region of hepatitis C virus : identification of a new virus type and restrictions on sequence diversity. J Gen Virol 1993 ; 74 : 661-8.
8. Okamoto H, Tokita H, Sakamoto M, Horikita M, Kojima M, Iizuka H, Mishiro S. Characterization of the genomic sequence of type V (or 3a) hepatitis C virus isolates and PCR primers for specific detection. J Gen Virol 1993 ; 74 : 2385.-90.
9. Simmonds P, Rose KA, Graham S, et al. Mapping of serotype-specific, immunodominant epitopes in the NS-4 region of hepatitis C virus (HCV) : use of type-specific peptides to serologically differentiate infections with HCV types 1, 2 and 3. J Clin Microbiol 1993 ; 31 : 1493-503.
10. Di Bisceglie AM, Martin P, Kassianides C, et al. Recombinant interferon alpha therapy for chronic hepatitis C. N Engl J Med 1989 ; 30 : 1506-10.
11. Davis GL, Balart LA, Schiff ER, et al. Treatment of chronic hepatitis C with recombinant interferon alpha. N Engl J Med 1989 ; 30 : 1501-6.
12. Kanai K, Kako M, Okamoto H. HCV genotypes in chronic hepatitis C and response to interferon. Lancet 1992 ; 339 : 1543.
13. Yoshioka K, Kakumu S, Wakita T, et al. Detection of hepatitis C virus by polymerase chain reaction and response to interferon-α therapy : relationship to genotypes of hepatitis C virus. Hepatology 1992 ; 16 : 293-9.
14. Takada N, Takase S, Enomoto N, Takada A, Date T. Clinical backgrounds of the patients having different types of hepatitis C virus genome. J Hepatol 1992 ; 14 : 35-40.
15. Pozzato G, Moretti M, Franzin F, Croce LS, Tiribelli C, Masayu T. Severity of liver disease with different hepatitis C viral clones. Lancet 1991 ; 338 : 509.
16. Weiner AJ, Kuo G, Bradley D, et al. Detection of hepatitis C viral sequences in non-A, non-B hepatitis. Lancet 1990 ; 335 : 1-3.
17. Kobayashi Y, Watanabe S, Konishi M, et al. Detection of hepatitis C virus RNA by nested polymerase chain reaction in sera of patients with chronic non-A, non-B hepatitis treated with interferon. J Hepatol 1992 ; 16 : 138-44.
18. Urdea MS. Synthesis and characterization of branched DNA (bDNA) for the direct and quantitative detection of CMV, HBV, HCV and HIV. Clin Chem 1993 ; 39 : 725-6.

Conclusion

S. ERLINGER

Service d'Hépatologie et Unité de Recherches de Physiopathologie Hépatique,
Hôpital Beaujon, Clichy, France.

Since the discovery of the hepatitis C virus in 1989, a considerable number of studies, clinical as well as molecular, has allowed to collect a lot of information on this virus. This workshop has permitted a survey of recent data.

The genetic variability of the virus has emerged rapidly after its discovery. C. Bréchot has pointed out the possible clinical implications. The viral RNA includes a 5' non coding region which is highly conserved and a region encoding for the enveloppe proteins, which is in contrast hypervariable. About 12 different genotypes have been individualized. The most frequent are genotypes I (or 1a), II (or 1b) and III (or 2a). It appears that genotype I (or 1b) is associated with an hepatic disease more severe, less recent and less sensitive to interferon than genotype I (or 1a). In a given population, several genotypes usually coexist. The determination of the genotype (and the quantification of viremia by molecular techniques) must be included in prospective studies of hepatitis C.

The quantification of viremia is also probably an important prognostic indicator. It was discussed by Thelu, Zarski and their coworkers. They indicate that, in their limited experience, viremia is better correlated with the response to alpha interferon than the genotype. This preliminary conclusion must be confirmed by larger studies.

The techniques of quantification are not yet standardized. The branched DNA method (Chiron) has been applied (together with genotyping) by Marcellin *et al.* to a population of 54 blood donors : 77 % of them had detectable viral RNA and the majority of them had genotype I or II. There was no correlation in this group between genotype and the importance of viremia and no correlation between viremia and serum aminotransferase activity. The accumulation and comparison of studies of this type will certainly allow a better understanding of the epidemiology of hepatitis C.

Other quantification methods using PCR have been presented by Wolfe *et al.* (Roche) and by Sillekens *et al.* (Organon). Similarly, as pointed out by the authors, larger studies are necessary to evaluate the prognostic value of viremia measured by these methods.

The gold standard of viremia is PCR. A great effort of standardization has been made between laboratories. J.J. Lefrère and the Groupe Français d'Études Moléculaires des Hépatites have clearly shown, with three successive panels of serum, that optimization and standardization of the technique were possible. Such quality control will be repeated and extended to genotyping and serotyping.

In daily practice, anti-HCV antibodies detected by Elisa and Riba are of the greatest diagnostic value. A frequent problem (in particular in blood donors) is the observation of an indeterminate result (with only one antibody positive out of the four included in the test). J.M. Pawlotsky has shown that, in blood donors, when aminotransferases are normal, an indeterminate test corresponds most ofte (albeit not always) to a negative viremia (by PCR). In contrast, in patients of specialized consultations, with an increased aminotransferase activity, an indeterminate test corresponds often to a positive viremia. In most cases, a third generation test (Riba 3) allows to solve the problem : a positive Riba 3 tests almost always indicates a positive viremia. However, some Riba 3 tests are still indeterminate.

L. Stuyver (Innogenetics) reviewed the genotyping methods : restriction fragment length polymorphism (RFLP) analysis, amplification with specific primers, or reverse hybridization. He presented preliminary results on European, Asian and African populations. We will know more on this in the near future.

Infection with hepatitis C virus is responsible of some extra-hepatic manifestations, often mediated by an immunological mechanism. Among these, cryoglobulinemia has attracted attention recently. F. Lunel and L. Musset have reviewed this fascinating area, together with their large personal experience. They confirm the role of the hepatitis C virus in the etiology of mixed cryoglobulinemia (previously referred to as « essential »). They find an infection with the hepatitis C virus in over 50 % of cases of mixed cryoglobulinemia, and, inversely, a cryoglobulinemia in approximately 50 % of cases of chronic virus C infection. In this case, viral RNA is found in the cryoprecipitate, an observation which suggests a role of the virus in the pathogenesis of cryoglobulinemia. Finally, the prevalence of cryoglobulinemia increases with the duration of the infection, and when there is cirrhosis. At this time, it is not yet possible to separate the role of time and that of the severity of the disease in the appearance of cryoglobulinemia.

In brief, this workshop is a superb illustration of the acceleration of progress induced by the tools of molecular biology. Five years after its discovery, much is known on the hepatitis C virus. There is still much to be done to understand the mechanisms of infection, the replication of this virus, to discover more efficient treatments, to imagine strategies for vaccination. No one is yet sure to have seen the virus. These are good reasons to look forward to future workshops.

Achevé d'imprimer par Corlet, Imprimeur, S.A.
14110 Condé-sur-Noireau (France)
N° d'Imprimeur : 4966 - Dépôt légal : août 1994
Imprimé en C.E.E.